THE FITNESS LEADER'S
EXERCISE BIBLE

Anterior View

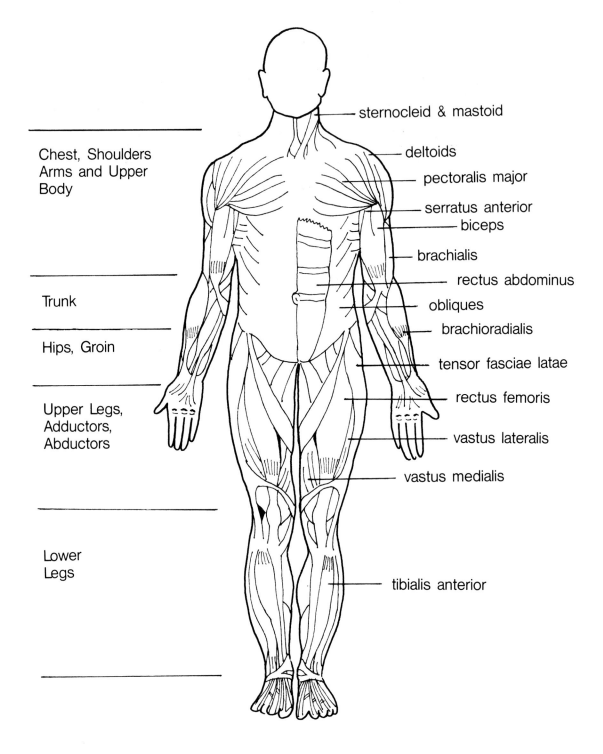

sternocleid & mastoid

deltoids

pectoralis major

serratus anterior

biceps

brachialis

rectus abdominus

obliques

brachioradialis

tensor fasciae latae

rectus femoris

vastus lateralis

vastus medialis

tibialis anterior

Chest, Shoulders
Arms and Upper
Body

Trunk

Hips, Groin

Upper Legs,
Adductors,
Abductors

Lower
Legs

Fig. 1

THE FITNESS LEADER'S EXERCISE BIBLE

Second Edition

Garry Egger Ph.D
Nigel Champion B.P.E.
Greg Hurst Dip. Health and P.E.

Companion Volume to the best selling
Fitness Leader's Handbook

Kangaroo Press

Posterior View

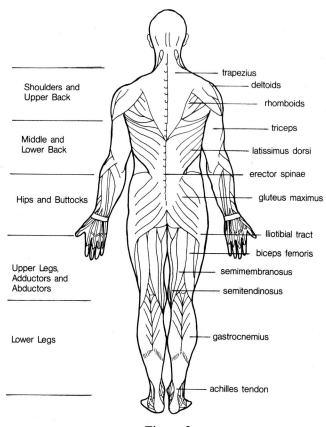

Shoulders and
Upper Back

Middle and
Lower Back

Hips and Buttocks

Upper Legs,
Adductors and
Abductors

Lower Legs

trapezius
deltoids
rhomboids
triceps
latissimus dorsi
erector spinae
gluteus maximus
lliotibial tract
biceps femoris
semimembranosus
semitendinosus
gastrocnemius
achilles tendon

Figure 2

Acknowledgments

Our thanks go to Suzie Miller of 'Suzie's Workout'
for modelling the exercises with Greg Hurst. Suzie
also gave great assistance with the decriptions for
the aerobic moves.

Reprinted 1990, 1991, 1992, 1993, 1994, 1995 and 1996
This revised edition first published in 1989 by Kangaroo Press Pty Ltd
3 Whitehall Road Kenthurst NSW 2156 Australia
P.O. Box 6125 Dural Delivery Centre NSW 2158
Printed in Singapore by Kyodo Printing Co (S'pore) Pte Ltd

ISBN 0 86417 260 5

Contents

Side Views

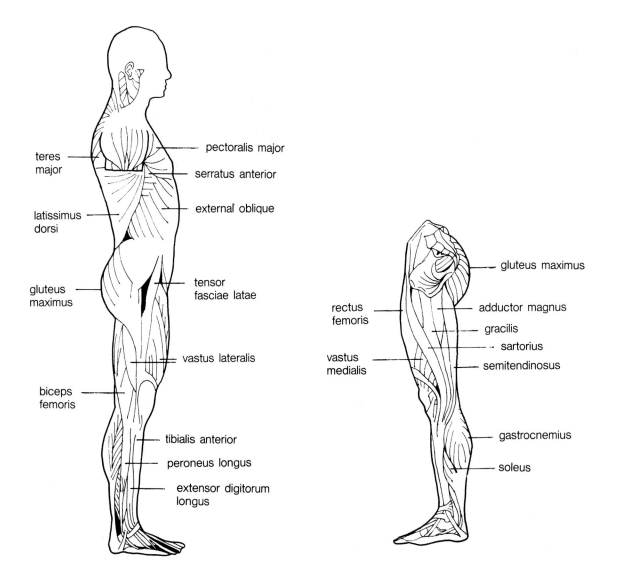

teres major

pectoralis major

serratus anterior

external oblique

latissimus dorsi

gluteus maximus

tensor fasciae latae

vastus lateralis

biceps femoris

tibialis anterior

peroneus longus

extensor digitorum longus

gluteus maximus

rectus femoris

adductor magnus

gracilis

sartorius

vastus medialis

semitendinosus

gastrocnemius

soleus

Figure 3

Introduction

1. The Fitness Revolution

Why do people exercise? This is a question often asked the wrong way around, i.e. why *don't* people exercise? Yet it seems more relevant to ask why thousands of people jog up and down the streets every day, beat a tennis ball relentlessly across a net, or risk being pounded into the sand by the surf. In other words, what has fuelled the modern fitness boom and how has this changed over the years?

The motivation to exercise is dynamic, not static. In the 1960s for example most people exercised for sport; in the 1970s for aerobic conditioning, and in the 1980s for cosmetic benefits.

Fitness books of the 1940s, few as they may have been, were primarily oriented towards equipping soldiers for war. The sergeant-major was the modern-day instructor, motivating through sheer terror, and motivating, of course, primarily males. Females were too delicate for such hard-core activities.

In the 1950s, the commercial gymnasium arose, but never really flourished. Universal Equipment manufactured the first resistance training systems, and American Joe Weider started his *Body Building* magazines gaining a small but dedicated following.

The 1960s is now thought of as an era of hedonism. Physical activity was generally restricted to those requiring fitness for sport. But a large proportion of the population chose not to exercise because they felt they had no need. Modern conveniences, for the first time in history, did most of the daily chores, and hence exercise, for them.

The upsurge in jogging in the 1970s arose largely out of a disillusionment with this type of lifestyle and the growing concern with heart disease that was presumed to be associated with such a sedentary existence. The simplest and easiest form of activity to combat this was, of course, jogging.

This was noticeable even in changes in the physique of the day—from increasing corpulence to that of the lean, trim and even emaciated morning, evening and afternoon jogger.

The introduction of exercise to music in the late 1970s and 1980s started a shift which is reflected in the aesthetics of the human body. Callisthenic exercises to music (aerobics) resulted in an overall physique which was less 'starved' looking than that of the runner. Also for the first time, it became obvious that women were interested in the suppleness of the male physique, just as men were interested in the hardening female body (in contrast to the soft, ample, Marilyn Monroe type figure of the 1950s). As a form of institutionalised exercise, aerobics has now become ingrained in modern society.

The renewed interest in physique has also resulted in a resurgence in one of the oldest forms of structured exercise—resistance or 'weight' training. Resistance training was said to have begun when the Greek god Milo carried a calf on his shoulders daily until it became a bull. Since then, weight lifting has become associated with masochism, machoism and 'muscleism'. But all that changed in the mid 1970s when film stars such as Bo Dereck and Jane Fonda showed that women were not prone to excessive muscle bulk as a result of resistance training. In fact, the resulting form was one of tight, firm muscle tone, on a trim, shapely body. Weight training in the 1980s became one of the fastest growing forms of physical conditioning of the day.

Underlying these changes has been a growing interest in exercise-induced injury—both acute and chronic. Because of the renewed interest in physical fitness and consequent rise in associated physiological research, huge strides have been made in correcting acute injuries through changes in form, type and intensity of exercise. Chronic and long-term injuries, on the other hand, continue to plague the regular exerciser. Like a motor car that is driven short distances, the human body seems capable of masking biomechanical difficulties when it is not physically stressed. But if the journey is longer, more regular and more intense, the chances of structural breakdown are increased enormously. The challenge is to reduce the incidence of such injury without reducing the efficiency of the exercise.

Flexibility training is now accepted as a useful form of injury prevention. The longer a muscle, the less chance of damage when that muscle is suddenly and dynamically taken to its full length. Flexibility is also now seen as important in its own right—as a necessary part of total body fitness. In order to function adequately in day-to-day life, a certain degree of flexibility is needed for bending, lifting, and preventing the muscle tightening caused by sedentary living.

Aerobics, weight training and flexibility then, are those forms of exercise which cover the fitness needs of the majority of the population. These will be categorised as *stamina*, *strength* and *suppleness*. As could be expected, a vast number of new and different exercises, and new and different ways of structuring exercises, have recently been discovered within each of these categories. Seldom however, have these been documented in a single, easily understood publication.

The Exercise Bible is intended to fill that gap. It was developed from years of experience in training fitness leaders through the Australian Council for Health, Physical Education and Recreation (ACHPER) program in Australia, and incorporating information from the highly successful 'Fitness Leader Exercise Encyclopedia Video' series, and is a companion to *The New Fitness Leader's Handbook*. It should be used in conjunction with the *Handbook* in order to gain a full understanding of exercise principles and practices. Although primarily written to service the needs of fitness leaders, *The Exercise Bible* is also intended for teachers, coaches, sportspeople and anyone interested in sport, exercise or fitness.

The book is divided into 3 sections, each with its own general introduction and background information. These are:

(a) Aerobic Floor Class Exercises
(b) Resistance Training Exercises
(c) Flexibility Exercises

Overall, there are some 600 exercises, either photographed or described. Where relevant, exercise progressions are described and incorrect and potentially dangerous exercises listed.

2. Basic Principles of Exercise

The first step in designing an exercise program is to establish a specific objective: to determine which physical parameters are to be improved. If body-weight and aerobic condition are important, aerobic exercise will be indicated; if muscle and joint stiffness is a problem, flexibility training should play a great part; if muscle strength is low, some strengthening work should be included.

Next, a program should be designed to meet the established objectives. This necessarily involves decisions about the *type*, *duration* and *frequency* of exercise as well as the means to evaluate progress in the form of relevant physiological and/or performance tests.

1. The training threshold

There is a minimum amount of exercise which is required to produce significant improvements in

any physical fitness parameter. This is referred to as the *training threshold*. For example, the recognised training threshold for the development of aerobic fitness in most people is regarded as 20 minutes of effort at a heart-rate of between 60% and 80% of maximum heart-rate (MHR).

2. Overload

Overload is a key concept in exercise programming. This implies that an individual must exercise at a level above that which can be normally carried out comfortably. For example, to increase the strength of a muscle, it must be contracted against a greater than normal resistance. The intensity, duration and frequency of exercise therefore, should be above the training threshold and should be gradually but progressively increased as the body adapts to the increased demands. As fitness levels improve, so the training threshold will be raised.

3. Specificity

The principle of *specificity* of training effects implies that different forms of exercise produce different results. The type of exercise carried out is specific both to the muscle groups being used and to the energy sources involved. For example, there is little *transfer of training* from strength training to the cardiovascular system. Similarly, prolonged running is unlikely to improve endurance swimming performances.

4. Reversibility

Training effects are reversible in that if workouts stop, or are not often enough or intense enough, loss of training can quickly occur. This can be prevented by continuing training at a maintenance level after a high level of conditioning has been obtained.

5. Progression

As a person becomes more fit, a higher intensity of exercise is required to create an overload and therefore provide continued improvements. This is most pertinent for athletes who wish not merely to maintain a good level of fitness but to improve on that level. Progression can be through either increased intensity or duration of exercise sessions.

6. Warm-up

Every exercise session should be preceded by a period of *warm-up* where the body is prepared gradually for the effort to come. Warm-up should be gentle and rhythmic and preferably use the muscles to be involved in the major activity. It should take up 10–20% of the time spent in the primary exercise.

7. Cool-down

As with the warm-up, a *cool-down* period should be a vital component of an exercise session. This involves a gradual decrease in the intensity of the exercise until the body's physiological functions return to the resting state. An adequate cool-down helps the muscles of the body return blood to the heart so that it does not pool in the muscles.

8. Frequency

To develop aerobic fitness, it has traditionally been taught that exercise should be carried out on a minimum of 3–4 days a week. However, this often leads to a grouping of exercise sessions early in the week. Hence a more appropriate protocol may be to ensure that exercise is not missed on 2 consecutive days.

During endurance training, total body mass and fat weight (FW) are reduced, while lean body mass (LBM) generally remains constant or increases slightly. Programs designed for fat loss should be carried out on a minimum of 3 days a week, for 20 minutes a time at an intensity designed to expend approximately 13 200 kilojoules (300 calories). A similar effect can be gained with an energy expenditure of 8 800 kilojoules (200 calories) per session if the exercise frequency is at least 4 days per week.

In order to maintain a training effect, exercise must be carried out on a regular basis. There will be a significant reduction in fitness after 2 weeks of inactivity, with participants losing approximately 50% of their fitness after 4–12 weeks and 100% after 10–30 weeks.

9. Intensity

Because heart-rate increases linearly with effort, this is often used as a measure of the required intensity of exercise. A training effect is gained if the exercise heart-rate is maintained at a rate between 70–85% of the maximum heart-rate (MHR) where MHR is determined by the formula: MHR = 220 − age.

Another simple test of intensity is to ensure that the exercise pulse reaches a count of 120–130 beats per minute during exercise. This sets a safe lower value for the establishment of a training effect at most ages. At a higher level, the 'talk test' can be used to assess whether an individual is working out too hard. If the exerciser cannot comfortably talk (or whistle) while exercising, the effort is more than likely anaerobic and therefore of greater intensity than necessary for safe training. For beginners it is unwise to continue at this level.

10. Duration

The minimum length of time of an exercise session for aerobic benefit is 15–20 minutes. Improved performance will continue (within reason) the longer the exercise session is continued. Beyond an hour, the returns start to become less. It is at this level that one might train if competition is the desired end.

For a beginning exerciser, it is often unwise to continue an exercise session beyond 30 minutes at the intensity prescribed above. Sessions should be limited to 15–20 minutes. If necessary, recovery periods of 1–2 minutes can be included between the heavier segments of activity.

Part A: Aerobic Floor Class Exercises

Background

Aerobics to music was virtually unknown in the 1970s. However in recent years it has become one of the most popular forms of exercise, rivalling jogging for popularity.

The word 'aerobic' has been used for years in the scientific world to describe the form of metabolism involving energy liberated in a muscle in the presence of oxygen. However the term 'aerobics' has become synonymous in the public mind with exercise to music (a version of which has been called 'aerobic dance').

The increase in interest is well deserved. A good aerobics program can improve aspects of aerobic conditioning, flexibility, strength and agility, as well as provide a safe and sociable form of exercise.

1.1 The Structure of an Aerobics Class

An aerobics class should be similar in structure to other aerobic fitness programs. There should be 3 phases: warm-up, conditioning, and cool-down.

The Warm-Up Phase: The purpose of the warm-up is to prepare the body for the following conditioning phase. There are 3 aspects to this preparation.

(i) *Warming the Body:* The prime function of this phase is to actually warm up. A general warming up can be achieved by using the major muscle groups in controlled, brisk, rhythmical activity. As energy is used, the elasticity of muscle tissue is increased, as is blood flow, thus enabling more oxygen and energy substrates to be carried to the parts of the body being worked.

(ii) *Mobility:* Many participants arrive at a class with limited mobility as they have been sitting at desks and in cars for most of the day. Normal mobility must be established in preparation for the conditioning phase. This can be achieved in conjunction with the warming up movements by ensuring all the joints are taken through a wide range of movement.

(iii) *Specific Stretching:* For some individuals such as the beginner or the injured exerciser, specific static stretching is recommended. The sites commonly needing attention for the beginner are the calf, hamstring, adductors, lower back and hip flexors. If exercising on a hard floor, calf stretching is particularly advisable. If high, straight-leg kicks are to be performed, hamstring stretching is warranted. Considerations for the instructor when determining the need for static stretching in the warm-up should be: the participants, the environment and the exercises to be performed. These stretches can either be held for several seconds or slowly and rhythmically moved into and out of the end of range of motion.

The Conditioning Phase: This is obviously the most important phase of the class. Vigorous movements provide the 'overload' needed for improvement and the instructor would normally include an aerobic and a strength component in the standard class.

(i) The aerobic component is aimed at improving the capacity of the body to deliver and use oxygen in the working muscles. To do this, the class should be sufficiently intense for participants to reach a working heart-rate of between 60% and 80% of maximum, for a duration of at least 15 minutes and preferably 20–30 minutes. The type of exercises selected should be those that incorporate large muscle groups; jumping, running, skipping, race walking and low-impact aerobic (LIA) steps are ideal. Intensity can be increased by using the arms in co-ordination with the legs.

(ii) The strength component comes from exercises involving resistance through gravity, body weight, a partner and equipment such as hand weights and rubber bands.

The Cool-Down Phase: This phase represents a tapering-off period after the completion of the main workout. The aim is to return the body to a steady state. There are two aspects to this phase.

(i) Recovering after the conditioning phase is best accomplished by a continuation of the conditioning phase at a decreasing intensity. This can be carried out by performing rhythmical movements similar to the warm-up or by isolation floor exercises. The intensity should decrease to a point where the participants are only working on flexibility and relaxation exercises.

(ii) Flexibility development is essential at the conclusion of a class. Stretches should be held for at least ten seconds.

1.2 Golden Rules for Aerobics Instruction

There are 5 basic rules that should form the basis of every good aerobics class:

1. Safety

Before anything else, a class must be safe. This means protection against both chronic and acute injuries, and involves paying special attention to:

Screening: While gentle and progressive exercise is safe for most people, there are those who may overstress themselves in a large class where close supervision is difficult. If injury occurs to such an individual there may be cause for litigation against an instructor if correct screening procedures have not been adopted.

To prevent this, all class participants should be screened to identify pregnant females, diabetics, those who have been habitually inactive and those with a history of heart disease or with high heart-disease risk (i.e. due to blood pressure, smoking, or overweight).

Exercise Format: When one part of the body is continually stressed, chronic injuries can occur. The most common problem in the aerobics class is lower leg injuries due to continuous high-impact moves such as jumping and running. Injuries can be prevented without sacrificing the aerobic benefits, by incorporating low-impact moves. This alternating between high-impact and low-impact moves keeps the heart-rate high while stress is reduced on the lower leg.

The older style of 'go for the burn' type aerobics is obsolete and in many instances contraindicated in the modern aerobics class. Repeating a movement to exhaustion can lead to physiological damage as well as demotivation, since the average person does not enjoy being continually subjected to failure. A class is truly successful when the participants complete all movements while at the same time getting a good workout.

Environment: (a) *Floor Surface:* Incorrect floor surfaces are commonly linked with lower leg injuries. For maximum protection, a floor surface must be shock absorbing but not so soft as to provide inadequate stability. Friction between the shoe and foot must also be sufficient to allow a grip, but not so excessive as to prevent some movement of the foot.

The table, adapted from the National Injury Prevention Foundation, shows the advantages and disadvantages of various common floor surfaces.

(b) *Footwear:* Good footwear in an aerobics class is vital. Well cushioned shoes providing stability and correct movement dramatically reduce lower leg and back injuries. Choosing the correct shoe however is a little more difficult because there is no one shoe that suits all. The effectiveness of a shoe will depend on the person wearing it and the mode of exercise.

In general, a shoe intended for aerobics should provide the following:

i Heel and forefoot stablity.

ii Forefoot and rearfoot shock absorption.

iii A sole surface that grips the floor to avoid slip but will not catch when turning.

iv Flexible in the mid and forefoot for easy flexion and extension, with lateral resilience to counter roll or twist.

v Adequate lacing for comfort and stability.

The best example of the ideal aerobic shoe can be found in the 'Reebok' aerobic range. Reebok pioneered the development of specialist aerobic

Floor Surface Characteristics

Surface	Impact Absorption	Stability Control	Friction With Shoes	General Comments
concrete/asphalt	very poor	excellent	very good	Not recommended
concrete with carpet	very poor	excellent	good	Worse than concrete—feels cushioned but is not
wood on concrete	very poor	excellent	good	As above
carpet on padding on hard surface	depends on padding	depends on padding	good	Acceptable if right amount of padding
gym mats	excellent	very poor	good	problems with ankle instability
sprung wooden floor	good	good	good	Good compromise for most situations
sprung wood with carpet and light under-cushion	very good	good	good	Perhaps the best combination

shoes and they lead the world in research, design and performance.

Irrespective of the brand, *well cushioned supportive footwear should be worn in all exercise classes.*

(c) *Ventilation:* Exercise in high temperature can lead to heat exhaustion, heat stroke and possibly death. It is important therefore that temperature and humidity be controlled through either adequate natural ventilation, fans or air conditioning in hot summer months. Although cold conditions are often uncomfortable for exercise, most research shows that hot, humid conditions pose more of a threat to health than cold, dry weather.

As a general guide, vigorous activity should not be carried out (particularly in heat unacclimatised individuals) in temperatures above 30 degrees centigrade when the humidity is greater than 70%.

(d) *Hydration:* Water should be available to exercisers at all times and they should be encouraged to drink particularly in hot conditions.

Space Allowance: Different types of classes require different amount of space. Running in a confined space for example is dangerous because of the damage to knees and ankles that can be caused by running around tight curves. A 'stretchercise' class on the other hand, may require less space because there's little movement from the one position.

For this reason it's difficult to categorically define floor space area required. The NSW Fitness Industry Association (FIA) suggests an average floor space area in floor classes of 3 square metres per person. However, recommendations put to the Australian Fitness Accreditation Council (AFAC) suggest a minimum floor space area of 5 square metres (i.e. roughly 2.2 × 2.2 metres).

Safe Exercise Selection: This means avoiding or substituting for exercising which may be potentially dangerous. A number of these, as well as errors in the instructors form, have been identified and are discussed later in the chapter.

2. Simplicity

Whilst exercise physiology is a complex subject, exercise practice should be simple. In general, conducting an exercise class should be like writing a report; if one simple word has the same impact as two difficult words, the former should always be preferred.

If a movement is simple, effective and fun, there's no reason why it should be sacrificed for another, more complex movement. If a movement is simple, form mistakes are less common and hence there is less chance of injury. If a movement is simple, participants are less likely to become frustrated and hence unable to mentally commit themselves to the movement.

3. Effectiveness

A good class should be designed specifically to achieve the desired goals. An Instructor should therefore determine whether the purpose is e.g. strength, tone, shape, fat loss etc. The class format then needs to be designed accordingly and appropriate exercises selected.

Strength exercises require assistance, either in the form of calisthenics (i.e. body weight), or resistance equipment. Toning and shaping classes need extended effort to burn fat as well as specific work to tone muscle. Fat loss classes call for extended aerobic activity.

Much time and effort is wasted in floor classes carrying out ineffective and uneconomic movements. Apart from filling in time, these have little value and some possible potential danger in an exercise class. Effectiveness may sound a logical criterion for exercise selection, but the principle is not always adhered to in practice.

4. Variety

It's an old cliché, but in an aerobics class, variety really IS the spice of life. As in most other aspects of life, stimulation is needed to maintain interest in any particular form of repetitive behaviour. Aerobic floor classes are one form of aerobic exercise, and as such will tend to wax and wane in popularity as other forms of exercise develop. Within an aerobic floor class, the interest can be stimulated by varying exercises, music, format, intensity and style of the class.

Recent developments in floor classes include the use of:
- circuits in the class
- large rubber bands and hand weights
- organised action e.g. lines, circles etc.

- varying class structures e.g. multi-peaking, single peak and reverse peak.

5. Enjoyment

Finally, for an individual to adhere to an exercise program it has to be enjoyable. This means creating an atmosphere through the quality of instruction, as well as attention to all the above golden rules.

Applying Scientific principles to the Aerobics Class

Whilst knowledge about exercise has increased enormously in recent years, there is often a lack of cross-fertilisation from one branch of sport or exercise to another. Strength training and body building for example, are areas where dedicated research and practice has resulted in improvements in knowledge about exercise efficiency and technique. Some of the findings from these fields can be utilised in planning the aerobic floor class. For example:

1.3 Aerobic Exercises NOT Recommended

Successful litigation against Jane Fonda for her exercise tapes and injury to individuals in home exercise programs, has led to a greater awareness of injury risks from incorrect exercises. Yet in many cases, researchers only identify dangerous exercises after the damage has been done. And with increasing numbers now exercising, the list is growing.

The 'no-no' list published below gives a three star rating for a variety of *not* recommended exercises based on inefficiency and/or danger to *non-elite athlete* clients. The rating key is:
* Inefficient/dangerous if done incorrectly
** potentially dangerous
*** potentially very dangerous

1. Neck rotations (**) (fig. 1):
Can cause neck damage if carried out too quickly, particularly the posterior portion of the movement. Excessive hyperextension of the neck should be avoided at all times.
Alternative: **Controlled linear movements:** Turn to the left then right then forward then back alternately, in a controlled manner.

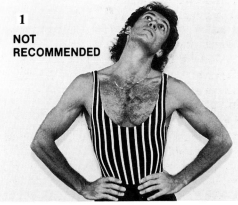

1 NOT RECOMMENDED

2. Straight-leg sit-ups (**) (fig. 2):
Potentially dangerous for the lower back for 3 reasons: (a) due to intervertebral compression the discs between the vertebrae are subjected to very high pressure, (b) the abdominals may not be strong enough to maintain the integrity of the lower back. The resulting hyperextension can lead to disc and ligament damage, and (c) a common cause of lower back injury is the muscular imbalance arising from strong hip flexors in

relation to weak abdominals. The straight-leg sit-up emphasises the hip flexors promoting this imbalance. Although contraindicated for the average participant some individuals may have a specific reason to strongly work hip flexors e.g. sprinters and ballet dancers.

Alternative: **Flexed-hip sit-ups** (*see* page 24).

3. Straight-leg raises (***) (fig. 3):
As for 2, except that the potential danger in lower back is greater.
Alternative: **Flexed-hip leg raises:** Bring bent knees to chest and return.

4. Straight-leg scissors/flutter kicks (***) (fig. 4):
As for 2. Potentially dangerous for the lower back as well as inefficient.
Alternative: **Flexed-hip scissor kicks/flutters:** Carried out with thighs perpendicular to floor, knees at right angles.

5. Hyperextension of back (***) (fig. 5):
Can put pressure on a weak lower back, particularly by raising arms and legs together from the prone lying position.
Alternative: **Alternate arm/leg raise:** While still in the prone position, raise alternate arm and leg or arms/legs separately.

6. Forced hyperextension (***) (fig. 6):
If the hips are allowed to sag towards the floor from the push-up position, gravity forces the lower back into a compromising position. The resulting intervertebral compression and ligament strain can be damaging.
Alternative: **Sphinx stretch:** Lie on the stomach with the elbows pulled in close to the side. Slowly raise onto the elbows as far as is comfortable and hold.

7. High hip leg extension on hands and knees (***) (fig. 7):
The back is put into hyperextension by forcefully kicking up with a straight leg, particularly while on the hands and knees.
Alternative: **Controlled leg extension on elbows:** By resting on the elbows the hips are angled down allowing a greater and more stabilised range of movement. Adbominals should be contracted to flatten the back. Lift the leg backwards in a controlled manner and the gluteals can be worked effectively without compromising the lower back.

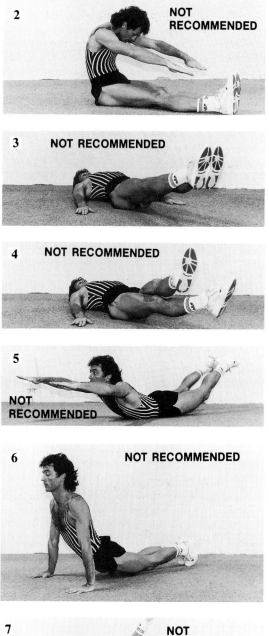

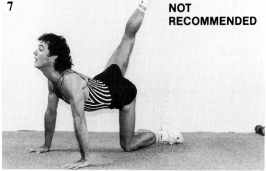

8. Rapid toe touching with bounce (***) (fig. 8):
Ballistic movements in the toe-touching position can cause lower back damage.
Alternative: **Sit and reach:** Sitting on the floor takes the gravitational effect out of the action. Reach forward slowly without bouncing to hold a stretch.

9. Deep squats (**) (fig. 9):
Can cause ligament damage in the knee as well as aggravation to the patella, particularly in the novice. This movement earns a 3 star rating if done quickly. All participants, including the elite should avoid 'bottoming out' in a squat. Other exercises which may have similar dangers for the knees are Rotated Knees as in a 'Skiers Movement' (fig. 9a) and the duck waddle (fig. 9b).
Alternative: **Half squats:** Pressure on the knee joint increases by up to 7-fold beyond the position of thighs parallel to the floor. Hence stopping before parallel essentially eliminates the problem.

10. Hurdler's stretch (***) (fig. 10):
Dangerous when the bent leg is turned out away from the body such that the medial and cruciate ligaments of the knee are twisted unnaturally.
Alternative: **Hurdler's stretch with bent leg tucked under:** Emphasis is taken off the knee with the bent leg tucked under the buttocks or if the leg is bent around to the front.

11. Long arm circles (*) (fig. 11):
According to some physicians, there is a potential danger to the shoulder tendons and nerves when the arms are held horizontally (in a long lever position) and repeatedly moved through a small range of movement. As well as being potentially dangerous the movement is grossly inefficient.
Alternative: **Large range of motion:** This works the deltoids through their full range of motion without impingeing on nerves and tendons in the shoulder joint.

12. Jumping too fast/too slow/on toes/with straight knees (**) (fig. 12):
Can cause damage to lower limbs, particularly shin splints.
Alternative: **Correct speed/ground the heel:** The speed of jumping and running movements should be slow enough so that the heel can be properly grounded allowing the foot to be used correctly, while being fast enough for the movement not to be laboured, particularly in kicks and runs.

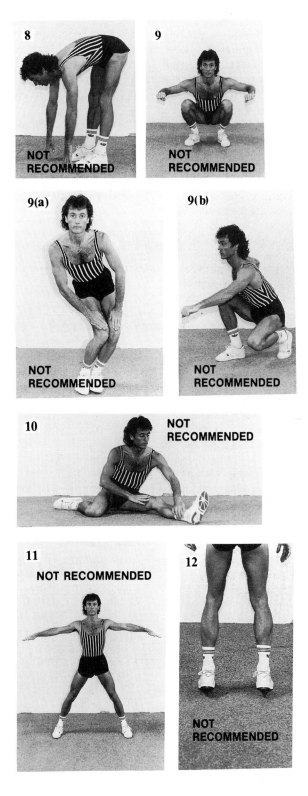

13. Running in the same direction (*) (fig. 13):
The lateral stress of running around corners, repeatedly, in the same direction, can lead to lower-leg injuries.
Alternative: **Varying running direction:** Alternate direction of running frequently.

14. Legs over head stretch (***) (Fig. 14):
While lying on back, take straight legs over the head until the feet touch the floor. The aim of the move is to stretch the upper back and neck but the neck is abnormally stressed as the entire body-weight is balanced in that area. The position is also unstable and a novice will commonly perform the move incorrectly.
Alternative: **Seated upper back stretch:** Sit with the legs crossed in front and bend the back forwards. By pulling up with the hands under crossed legs the stretch can be increased.

15. Seated quadricep stretch (**) (fig. 15):
Carried out by sitting back between the heels. This takes the knee joint out of alignment and hyperflexes the joint, leading to potential knee damage.
Alternative: **Standing quadricep stretch:** In standing position pull the foot back and up towards the buttocks and hold. Avoid hyperextension of the back by contracting the stomach muscles thus flattening the back.

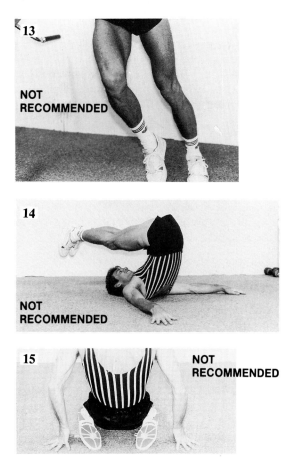

1.4 Common Errors of Form in Aerobics Classes

The ideal fitness class is characterised not just by *what is done* but by *how it is done*. In some situations an effective exercise can be made ineffective, and even dangerous, by simple changes to the pattern or shape of the movement. Varying the angle of joints and the position of limbs alters the stress on the muscle or joint. In some cases this may not be desirable.

The exercises listed below are those where common errors of form are made. Often, form becomes gradually worse with fatigue. Hence, the fitness leader should be constantly aware of the level of effort involved by class participants and the effects of this on form.

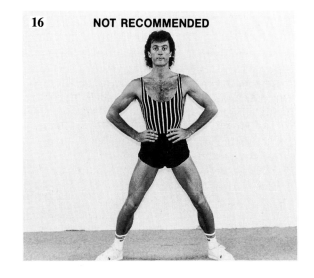

1. Squatting with inverted knees (fig. 16):
The knee is a hinge joint and as such is designed to move in only one plane of movement. The knee joint can be injured if it does not track correctly

during any type of knee bend. It is common, particularly in women for the knees to roll inwards during squatting and lungeing. The direction the knee joint should take is determined by the direction the feet are pointing. The knee should bend out and over the foot in the same direction as the toes.

2. Bending to side in side leg raise (fig. 17):
While on the knees and raising one leg to the side in the 'Rover' position, ensure the stabilising leg is kept perpendicular to the floor and body is not twisted with the action. This is a common mistake made when fatigued. The instructor should be sensitive to this problem and not push the participants into local muscle exhaustion.

3. Rotation of hips in waist twisting (fig. 18):
Side twisting in the standing position is meant to work the obliques, which are only mobilised if the hips and lower limbs remain locked. Ensure twisting does not include the lower body as this places rotational stress on the knee joint. The movement should not be exaggerated, particularly at speed as this compromises the lower back.

4. Locked knees in bent-over position (fig. 19):
When the legs are kept straight while flexing forwards at the hips a great deal of pressure is placed on the lower back. Most movements should not exceed 30 degrees flexion at the hips and the legs should always remain bent to distribute the load.

5. Forwards flexion and rotation (fig. 20):
Any movement involving rotation while flexing forwards at the hips while standing, should be avoided. Whether the legs are bent or not the stress on the lower back is too high.

6. Sit-ups with neck hyperextension (fig. 21):
In the sit-up position the chin should be kept in a neutral position. When the jaw is pushed up and out, the neck is hyperextended and if the chin is pulled in too tight it is hard to breathe.

7. Hyperextension of the back with extended arms (fig. 22):
If the arms are thown back in an extended position the back may tend to arch putting excessive pressure on the lower and middle back. This is also the case if the arms are extended above the head. The problem can be corrected by using bent arms in the movement.

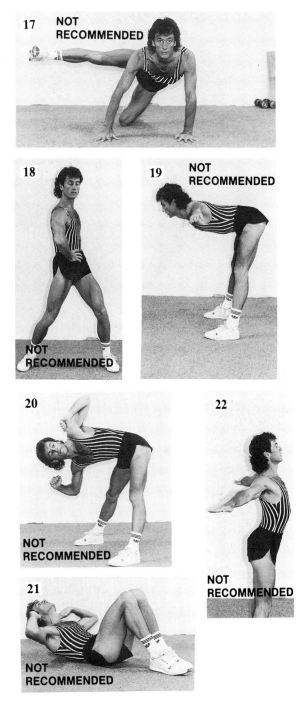

8. Rotated supporting knee (fig. 23):
Where the body is twisted and support is thrown onto a twisted knee, excessive rotational pressure is placed on the ligaments of the knee. This should be avoided by ensuring the knee is aligned over the foot and points in the same direction.

9. Back hyperextension in the 'all-fours' position (fig. 24):
Ensure that the back is not allowed to sag when working on all fours. All effort should be made to keep the lower back level.

10. Back of the hands together at the top of a long arm movement (fig. 25):
If the arms are moved in a full arc from below the body to above the head, the shoulder joint is restricted if the palms are turned out at the top of the movement. This puts excessive pressure on the shoulders and could lead to joint problems. Turn the palms to the front or inwards, once the arms move above shoulder height.

11. Ballistic kicking (fig. 26):
High kicks can be dangerous because of the ballistic action required to raise the leg to its full height. The temptation to kick high should be avoided, the leg should only be raised as far as is comfortable.

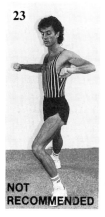

23 NOT RECOMMENDED

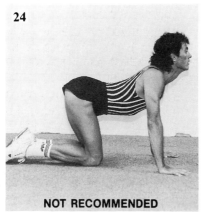

24 NOT RECOMMENDED

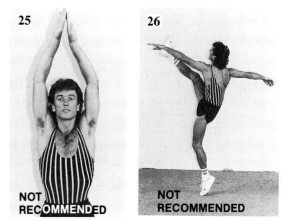

25 NOT RECOMMENDED

26 NOT RECOMMENDED

1.5 Music

Good music is the lifeblood of an aerobics class. Music should be carefully selected under the following guidelines:

Tempo: Finding the correct tempo is the hardest aspect of music selection. There is usually plenty of warm-up, cool-down and floor music, as this is used for dancing, but jumping and running music is always hard to find. By using a variable speed turntable, many tracks that would normally be too slow can be speeded up and used for the aerobic moves. The following breakdown details the speeds common used for different sections of an aerobics class:

- Warm-up: 124–136 beats/min.
- Jump: 140–150 beats/min.
- Run: 160–180 beats/min.
- Slow floor (abdominals and long lever work): 110–124 beats/min.
- Fast floor (chest, arms, back and short lever work): 120–132 beats/min.
- LIA travelling: 128–138 beats/min.
  [see page 37]
- LIA (stationary): 140–150 beats/min.

Popularity: Music should be chosen not only to personal preference. Participant's likes and dislikes should also be considered by using a variety of styles. Avoid anything that has offensive language or sounds 'noisy'.

Motivating: Music needs to be positive. Energetic, happy numbers are always better than depressing ballads. The mood of the music should suit the movements e.g. chose exciting, lively music for aerobic moves, but relaxing soothing music for cool-downs.

Consistency: Many tunes may sound great, but are less than effective if the tempo changes or the tune misses some beats throughout. Consistent music enables concentration on the class and not the music.

Quality: Much time and money can be spent on finding good music but if the quality of the recording or the sound system is substandard, all efforts could be wasted. Good quality tapes and recording facilities should be used and the system should be regularly cleaned and serviced.

1.6 Guidelines for Conducting Aerobics Classes

The following are guidelines for the running of aerobic floor classes as developed by the Australian Fitness Accreditation Council (AFAC).

1. The session must have a genuine aerobic component which lasts for a minimum of 15 minutes at an intensity measured preferably by:

(a) a minimum heart-rate of 120 beats per minute, or

(b) a heart-rate range defined by the formula 60–80% max heart-rate—age.

2. Clients should be encouraged to carry out such exercise at least 3 times per week.

3. There must be at least 5 minutes spent warming-up and mobilising at the start of the program and 5 minutes spent in slow stretching and cooling down at the end.

4. Stretching must be static, Proprioceptive Neuromuscular Facilitation (PNF), or gentle Range of Motion (ROM) type—particularly if participants in a group are beginning exercisers.

5. Stretching must include the major muscle groups to be used in the aerobic exercise to follow.

6. Progression from warm-up to aerobic effort must be gradual as it should also be with cool-down.

7. Ballistic movements should be avoided as much as possible during the progression of the program, particularly for inexperienced exercisers.

8. As far as possible, classes should be structured to cater for beginning and advanced exercisers, with separate classes conducted for each.

9. There should be approximately 4 m² of floor space per person in classes involving callisthenics or aerobic exercise to music.

10. All new participants in a class should be screened as to their exercise history, physical limitations, predisposition to injury and risk of heart disease, and advised as to the level recommended for their purpose.

11. Exercises involving hyperextension of the lower back must be avoided particularly for beginning classes.

12. Attention must be given to the correct procedures in carrying out specific exercises.

13. Advice should be given to certain clients about the level of difficulty of some exercises i.e. many men may have difficulty with certain flexibility exercises more suited to women (e.g. adductor/abductor stretches, back flexes etc.)

14. There should be no credence given to 'spot reduction' as a weight loss aid.

15. Advice should be given to clients on the appropriate clothing to be worn in classes.

16. If classes are carried out to music, this should be suitable to ensure a slow and gradual warm-up of at least 5 minutes and a similar cool-down.

17. Precautions must be taken at all times to prevent both acute and chronic injury.

18. Clients should be advised from the start of the program as to how long the class will be, and of any idiosyncrasies of the program that may not be expected.

19. There must be no scientifically unsupported promises made to clients regarding the expected benefits of an aerobic fitness class or aerobic exercise in general.

20. Clients must be asked if they are taking any form of medication, and if so what this may be. Where no knowledge about a medication is immediately available, steps should be taken to ascertain contra-indications of exercise, if any.

21. Clients should be advised to exercise before rather than after eating, but that limited fluid intake (with the exception of alcohol) before exercise is advisable.

22. Special attention should be paid to the possibility of dehydration in hot weather, particularly if exercise is carried out in the ambient environment. Advice should be given about fluid intake both before and after exercise.

23. All clients must be encouraged to wear well-cushioned and supportive shoes in classes involving running, skipping or hopping.

24. Clients must not be permitted to join classes after commencement when they may not have received sufficient warm-up.

25. Instructors must be aware of exercises regarded as potentially dangerous and which should be avoided or carried out with extreme care.

2. The Exercises

2.1 Exercises for the Upper Body

Standard exercise

1. The Push-Up: (fig. 27)
Uses: Develops strength in the pectorals, triceps and anterior deltoid.
Description: Can be performed off the feet for advanced or from the knees for intermediate exercisers. Beginners can bring their knees even closer to their hands to shorten the lever and therefore make the exercise easier. Hands positioned slightly more than shoulder width apart. Bend arms so that the chest almost touches the ground and then push to straighten the arms completely.

Special considerations
• The body must be kept straight. If the hips sag forwards the lower back will be stressed.

Variations
• **Narrow/Wide Push-Ups** (fig. 28). The wide position emphasises the chest and the narrow position concentrates more on the triceps. Both can be performed off the knees either repeatedly in the same position or alternately wide and narrow. Only the wide position should be used off the feet. A variation of the narrow push-up can be seen in fig. 29. Here the hands are pointing to the front with the thumbs next to each other. This brings the elbows closer together and places a greater load on the triceps. Another advanced push-up variation can be seen in fig. 30. Here the elbows are kept close to the sides with the hands pointing forwards.

• **Staggered push-up**, (fig. 31). Works the muscles of the shoulder at different angles. Perform off the toes for advanced, the knees for intermediate and bent body off the knees for beginners.

• **Side press**, (fig. 32). Emphasises the arm and chest on the same side as the press. This exercise can be repeated on the same side or roll and press to alternate sides. Suitable for all levels. To increase the workload wrap the bottom arm around the body (fig. 33).

• **One arm push-up**, (fig. 34). Overloads one side of the body at a time. The trunk is also used extensively as a stabiliser. With a straight body and the knees off the ground it becomes an advanced

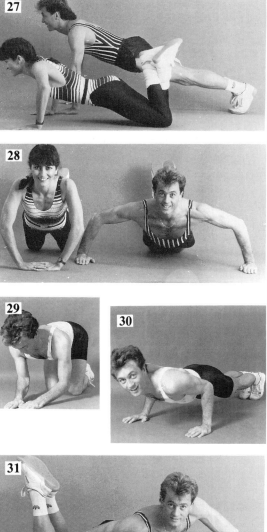

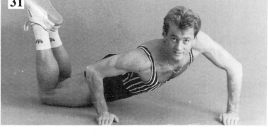

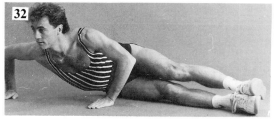

exercise. With a bent body position and the knees on the floor the exercise is suitable for intermediate and beginners.

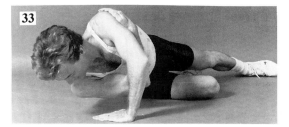

• **Rock back and press**, (Fig. 35). Rock back onto the heels then push forward for a press off the knees or the feet. Although the rock back does work the thighs and trunk, its main role is as an active rest between presses.

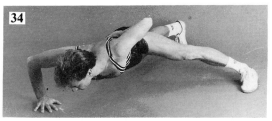

• **Clap push-up**, (fig. 36). Rock back as in figure 35, in moving forward towards the push up position clap the hands behind the back. For a more advanced exercise clap behind and in front (figure 37).

Note: When rocking back in figs 35 to 37 ensure that the movement is fluent and not ballistic. People with knee problems should avoid this exercise due to hyperflexion of the knee joint.

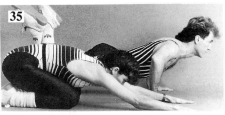

• **Reach through**, (fig. 38). In a bent body position on hands and knees, reach one arm between the opposite arm and knee. This works the back in rotation. By bending the supporting arm as in a push-up, the tricep and chest get a mild workout.

Other exercises

2. The dip: (fig. 39)

Uses: Prime movers are triceps and anterior deltoid. Most other shoulder muscles work to stabilise the joint in the movement.

Description: Weight is on the hands and feet with the back and buttocks straight and raised clear of the floor. Calves and arms should be vertical. Bend the arms to approximately 90 degrees then straighten.

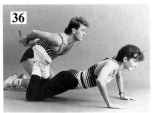

Special considerations:
• Preferably have the hands pointing forwards and the elbows backwards. This however can vary according to comfort.

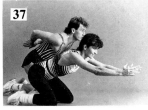

Variations:
• The load can be varied in the dip by changing the length of the lever. Those with weaker arms can leave the buttocks on the ground. Increase the load for the advanced by straightening the body (figure 40) or by taking one hand off the floor and wrapping it around the body (fig. 41).

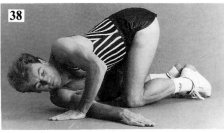

• For variety, perform the dip with one leg extended straight up or out (fig. 40), either repeatedly on the same side or use alternate legs. For beginners, separate the dip and leg extension into two movements and the leg extension becomes an active rest.

3. Isometric contractions:

Uses: An isometric contraction is a strong static

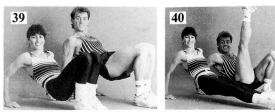

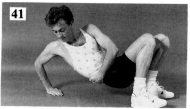

contraction where the joint angle does not change. It is hard to effectively exercise the biceps, lats and posterior deltoid in a floor class but isometrics can provide the resistance necessary.

Description: Using your own body as resistance contract as hard as is possible for a period of two to six seconds. To increase the energy cost, any of these exercises can be performed while squatting, lunging or jogging.

Special considerations:
• Due to the strength of the contraction blood pressure is easily raised and therefore these movements would not be appropriate for beginners.

Variations
• **Bicep curl,** (fig. 42). Grab the wrist in an overhand grip and curl up while pushing down. This will work the biceps and triceps of the opposite arm.
• **Lat pull** (fig. 43). Grasp both wrists in a monkey grip. Pull out and back to work the lattisimus dorsi.
• Hold a monkey grip behind the back (fig. 44) and pull out and up to work the deltoids or press the palms together behind the back to work the lats, biceps and rhomboids.
• Press the palms together (fig. 45) above the head

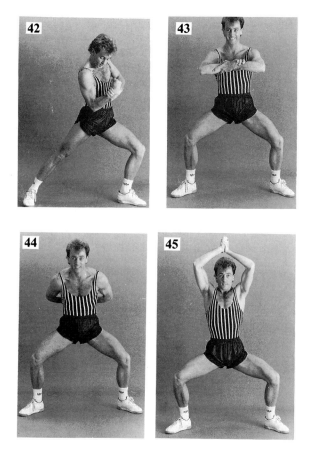

to work the upper pecs and trapezius. Pressing directly in front of the chest works the pecs and anterior deltoid.

2.2 Exercises for the Abdominals

Standard exercise

1. The Crunch: (fig. 46)
Uses: Works the rectus abdominus with assistance from the internal and external oblique muscles.
Description: Lie supine with the hips well flexed and the heels on the floor close to the buttocks. Arms can be in a variety of positions two of which are shown in fig. 46. Whatever position, do not throw the arms but keep them locked into a position so that the emphasis stays on the abdominals. The trunk should curl up to approximately 45 deg.

Special considerations:
• If the hips are not well flexed, the hip flexors will play a major role.

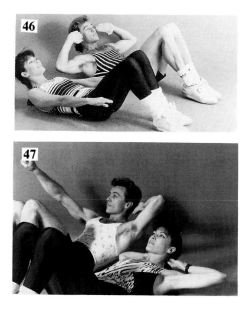

• Keep the head in a neutral position, if the neck is excessively flexed then breathing is difficult. If the neck is hyper-extended, neck injuries can occur. By maintaining a neutral position the common problem of discomfort at the base of the skull is reduced.

• Do not clasp the hands behind the head as the tendency is to pull on the head and stress the neck.

Variations

• Vary the arm positions by reaching forward with both arms and then with one arm (fig. 47) while the other supports the head.

• Simulate the action of pulling the body off the ground using an imaginary rope (fig. 48).

• Start by placing the hands by the side and while curling up flex the biceps to bring the forearms towards the face (fig. 49).

• Figs 50, 51 and 52 work the internal and external obliques as well as rectus abdominus. Flex the hips and with one foot off the floor bring the opposite elbow to touch the raised knee (fig. 50). Do a number of repetitions on one side before changing to the other side. Fig. 51 is a variation of fig. 50, but here, one leg is crossed over the other and the opposite elbow is raised to touch the knee. In fig. 52 both legs are raised off the ground in a flexed position. Place one arm out to the side to act as a stabiliser while the other reaches across the body to touch the outside of the opposite leg.

• Hips flexed with legs almost straight (fig. 53). Do not straighten the legs completely as many people, particularly men, do not have the flexibility to maintain this position comfortably.

• Have one leg raised and lift the upper body off the ground (fig. 54). Now bring into play the obliques by raising the opposite shoulder to the raised leg (fig. 55).

• **Oblique crunch,** (fig. 56). Roll bent legs to the side and crunch so that the external oblique of that side and the opposite internal oblique become the prime movers. Different arm positions can be used or reach to touch the foot.

2. The sit-up (fig. 57)

Uses: This exercise uses all the major abdominal muscles, rectus abdominus, external and internal obliques.

Description: Use the same starting position as the crunch. As the abdominal muscles are only capable of raising the trunk half-way, the arms must be used. This lowers the centre of gravity and adds momentum to the movement to get past the 'sticking point'. Start with the hands close to the chest and smoothly reach forward while sitting up.

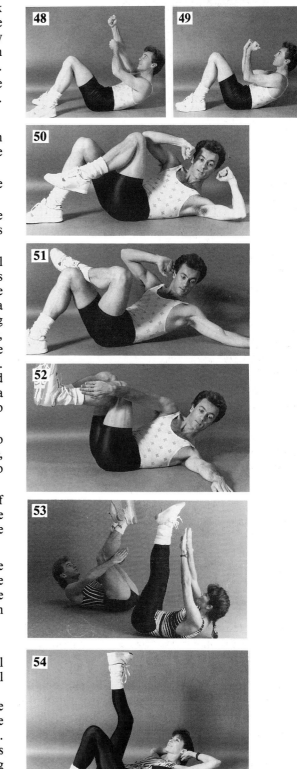

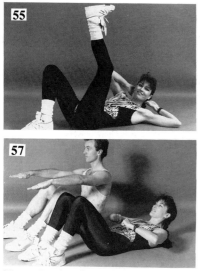

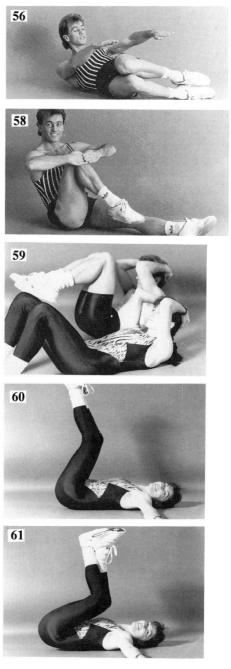

Note: In the sit-up when the trunk is raised more than 45 degrees off the ground the hip flexors become the primary muscles involved.

Special considerations
• Do not take straight arms back over the head when lying back down as this hyperextends the back.
• Be careful not to throw the arms but move them smoothly through the range of movement in concert with the abdominals. As the exerciser tires, the tendency will be to straighten the legs to incorporate hip flexors. This is ovbiously undesirable.
• Ensure that the full sit-up movement is fluent and that the 'V' position in the completion phase is not held.

Variations
• One leg bent, (fig. 58). One side of the hip always remains fully flexed. Repeat to the one side then change or bring the straight leg in while returning to the floor and extend the other leg out in the next sit-up. Do not extend both legs between sit-ups as the hip flexors will then play an even greater role.

3. Reverse abdominal curl (fig. 59)
Uses: This exercise works the inferior portion of the abdominals.
Description: Use the same starting position as the crunch. Instead of just raising the shoulders off the ground, bring the knees towards the chest (fig. 59).

Special considerations:
• The range of movement in the reverse curl is limited.
• Ensure the knees are bent and brought towards the chest.

Variations
• **Reverse curl with raised legs** (figs 60 and 61). Start with the legs crossed and raised (fig. 61). Now bring the knees towards the chest and raise the buttocks off the floor.

4. Double leg extension (fig. 62)
Uses: Safely exercises the hip flexors, and all the abdominal muscles.

Description: Sitting with both hands supporting the body, roll onto one hip with the knees drawn to the chest. Extend the legs (half-way for beginners and fully for intermediate and advanced), then pull the knees back into the chest.

Special considerations:
• Special care must be taken to keep the hips rotated to one side. If the exerciser lets the body straighten so that the hips are square the lower back can be stressed as the exercise becomes a double leg raise.

5. The bicycle (fig. 63)
Uses: Utilises all the muscles of the abdominal area and safely uses the hip flexors.
Description: Lie on the back with hands beside the head. Keep the shoulders lifted off the floor to maintain maximum abdominal involvement and alternately touch opposite knee and elbow. The more rotation in the movement the greater the load on the obliques.

Special considerations:
• A common mistake, particularly when tired, is to leave the shoulders on the floor. This not only means the abdominals are not being effectively worked, but also that the back can be hyperextended leading to back injuries.
• For beginners it would be best not to fully extend the legs.

Variations
• **Raised leg bicycle.** Start with one leg bent and

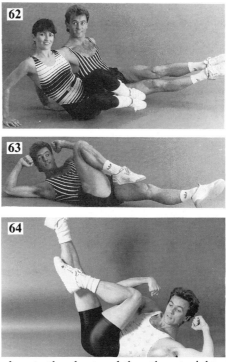

close to the chest and the other straight at an angle of about 70 degrees (fig. 64). Bring the elbow to the oposite knee and repeat on the other side.
• *Bent leg bicycle.* Start with the hips flexed and the feet close to the knee but keep the knee flexed when returning the foot to the floor.
• *Bicycle row.* Hold the knees with the hands. As the leg straightens, so too does the same arm.

2.3 Exercises for the Lower Back

Standard exercise

1. The back arch (fig. 65)
Uses: Strengthens all the postvertebral muscles of the back.
Description: Lie face down with the elbows bent and hands near the face. Lift the upper body off the floor while keeping the hips and the feet in contact with the floor. Lower the chest back down in a controlled manner.

Special considerations:
• It is essential that only the upper-body is lifted and the lower body remains in contact with the floor. This can be ensured by crossing the feet and pulling in tight with the buttocks.

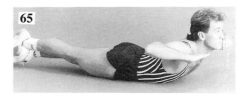

• It is not essential to lift as high as possible but rather lift as high as is comfortable.

Variations:
• Perform the standard exercise with the arms in different positions. By the side, at right angles to the body or clasping behind the back, (fig. 66). Do not reach the arms out to the front as this makes the lever unnecessarily long, therefore increasing intervertebral compression.

- Arch with a twist, (fig. 67). Slightly twist to alternate sides while extending the back.
- Clap behind the back or slap the buttocks as the back is extended.
- Reverse leg lift, (fig. 68). Reverse the body movement by keeping the upper body in contact with the floor and lifting the legs. For weak backs shorten the lever by bending the legs, (fig. 69) or raise one leg at a time (fig. 70).
- Opposite arm and leg, (fig. 71). Both the upper and lower body remain supported by keeping one leg and the opposite arm and chest on the floor. Alternate sides.
- Raise one side and twist, (fig. 72). As only one side of the body is being lifted and the lower body is supported, the arms can reach forward. The opposite can also be done for individual legs.
- Reach back and touch the foot, (fig. 73).

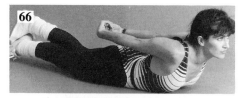

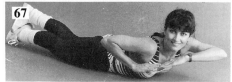

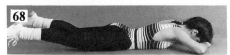

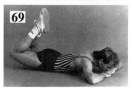

2. Back extension (fig. 74)

Uses: Strengthens postvertebral muscles of the back as well as hip extensors.

Description: Start supported on the hands and feet with buttocks just off the ground. Straighten the back until the body is flat.

Special considerations
- Do not hyper-extend the back.
- Ensure that the arms are kept straight.

Variations:
- Combine this movement with a dip to work the arms and shoulders with the back.
- Extend one leg out or up as the back is straightened. This movement can be repeated to alternate sides or alternated with a dip.

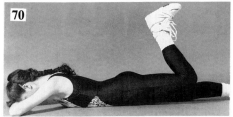

3. Back Press (Fig. 75)

Uses: Strengthens hip extensors and postvertebral muscles with emphasis on the lower back.

Description: Lie with back flat on the floor and feet close to the buttocks. Push the hips upwards to form a straight line from the shoulders to the knees. Keep the shoulders on the floor. Return towards the floor without touching before repeating.

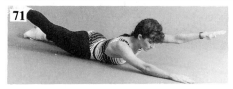

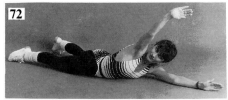

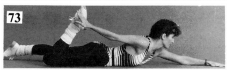

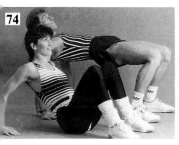

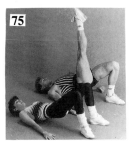

Variations:
- Extend a leg straight up and repeat to one side or alternate (fig. 75).
- Clap hands underneath the buttocks.
- Push the arms up similar to a bench press as the hips are raised.

Potentially dangerous back exercises

Double arch: (fig. 76)
The upper body and the lower body form two long levers with the lower back as the fulcrum. The muscular contraction required to lift both of these long levers simultaneously is so strong that the pressure on the back, in particular the intervertebral discs, can cause injury. It is really a case of the body being too strong for its own good. By shortening the levers or only lifting one end at a time the stress is reduced considerably.

Forced hyperextension: (fig. 77)
To lie prone and then push the body upwards can be safe provided the hips remain supported on the floor and the position is not uncomfortable. However, if the reverse occurs where the starting position is similar to that of a push-up and the hips are lowered towards the floor it is easy to dangerously hyperextend the lower back. Gravity

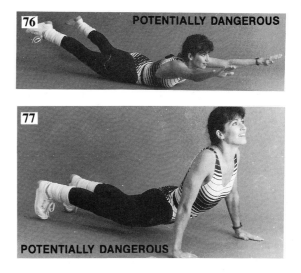

aggravates the problem by pushing the hips down and making it stressful to straighten back up.

2.4 Exercises for Hip Extensors, Abductors and Adductors

Standard exercise

1. Hip extension (Fig. 78)
Uses: Strengthens gluteus maximus and hamstrings.
Description: Start with the weight supported on both forearms and one knee, with the other leg extended behind. Raise the straight leg so that it is in line with the back. Bend the knee and lower the leg but do not let it touch the floor.

Special considerations:
• Do not raise the leg too high. Keep the movement controlled.
• Resting on the elbows angles the hips and back downwards so the range of movement is greater and the back is stabilised. However the back can still be dangerously hyperextended if the leg movement is not controlled.

Variations:
• **Bent leg hip extension.** Keep the knee bent at 90 degrees while lifting. As this shortens the lever it is ideal for beginners.
• **Extension kick.** Maintain a well supported flat back position. While keeping the thigh so that it is in line with the back flex the knee. This isometrically works the gluteals and dynamically works the hamstring.
• **Gluteal raise.** Maintain a well supported flat back

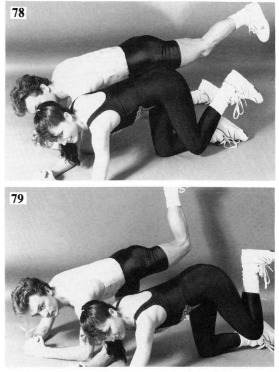

position. Start with the thigh being in line with the back, then lower the knee to the floor and raise back to the start position (fig. 79). This exercise is very good for working the gluteals.

- **Donkey kick**, (fig. 80). On hands and knees with the arms straight and the back flat, pull a knee into the chest and then push that leg straight out behind.
- **Combination donkey kick**, (fig. 81). Simultaneously reach and pull with the same arm as the leg being used.
- **Alternate donkey kicks** (fig. 82). Can be performed by touching the knee with the opposite hand.

Other exercises

2. Thigh lateral raise (fig. 83)
Uses: Strengthens the hip extensors and abductors.
Description: Adopt a hands and knees position with the back flat. Lift one bent leg out to the side then lower. Maintain a well supported position with the supporting thigh vertical. The range of movement should be approximately 45 degrees.
Variations:
- Lift the opposite supporting arm to the leg that is raised (fig. 84). Ensure that the body is well stabilised.
- **Lift and flick**, (fig 85). Start with the leg bent but as the thigh is laterally raised to 45 degrees straighten the leg. Bend the knee when lowering to return to the original position. As the lever lengthens, the resistance is greater.
- **Side kick**, (fig. 86). Start in the same position as fig. 85 and extend the leg laterally. It is not advisable to lift the leg off the ground when it is extended out to the side.
- **Rotational lateral leg raise.** This is similar to the standard high lateral raise except that the thigh is circled backwards as it is lifted and forwards as it is lowered.

3. Side leg raise (fig. 87)
Uses: Isolates and strengthens the abductors of the thigh, particularly gluteus medius and minimus.
Description: Lie on the side supported on the forearm, with the body in a straight line from head to toe. Lift the leg to about 40 cms and when lowering it ensure that it does not touch the bottom leg.

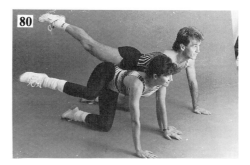

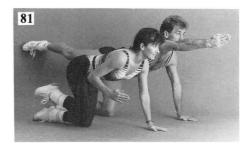

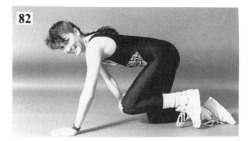

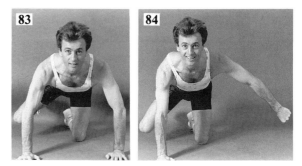

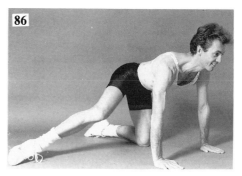

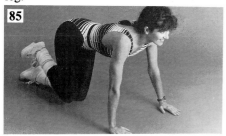

Special considerations:

• Do not raise the thigh too high.

• If the thigh turns out as it is lifted, the hip flexors become the prime movers and not the abductors. To avoid this keep the free arm in front of the body so the body does not roll back, flex the foot and concentrate on keeping this horizontal. If the flexed foot points up even slightly the emphasis moves to the hip flexors. The range of movement is not great and most people will only lift 30–45 degrees.

Variations:

• Roll the body slightly forward and rest on both elbows while performing a side leg raise. This will bring the gluteus maximus into play assisting the medius and minimus.

• Keep the leg being lifted bent to shorten the lever as shown in fig. 88. This reduces the resistance and is therefore ideal for beginners.

• Place the head on the arm and the bottom leg bent, raise the top leg as shown in fig. 89. Or, support the head on the hand (fig. 90).

• In order to increase the load raise the hips off the ground as shown in fig. 91.

• **Frontal side leg raise,** (fig. 92). Bend the thigh and the knee at 90 degrees. Take the free arm to the back to balance. Raise up and down through 45 degrees. Any higher than this and the hip flexors become the prime movers. Beginners should keep the leg bent. More advanced exercisers can straighten the knee to increase the load.

• **Side leg kick.** The starting position is that shown in fig. 92. Instead of lifting, simply straighten and bend the leg while keeping the thigh bent at 90 degrees.

• Start in the position shown in fig. 87 with the top leg slightly raised. Instead of lifting the leg, take the straight leg forward until the thigh is at 90 degrees to the body, then extend the thigh behind the body.

• **Abductor circles.** Similar to the standard side leg raise except circle the thigh forward as it is lifted and back as it is lowered.

4. Inner thigh raise (fig. 93)

Uses: Strengthens the adductor muscles of the inner thigh.

Description: Lie on the side supported by the lower forearm and the body in a straight line from head to toe. Cross the top leg over the bottom leg and place the foot on the floor next to the bottom knee. Grasp the ankle for stablity. Lift the thigh up as high as possible without rotating the thigh inwards.

Special considerations:

• Do not roll the body to the back and/or rotate

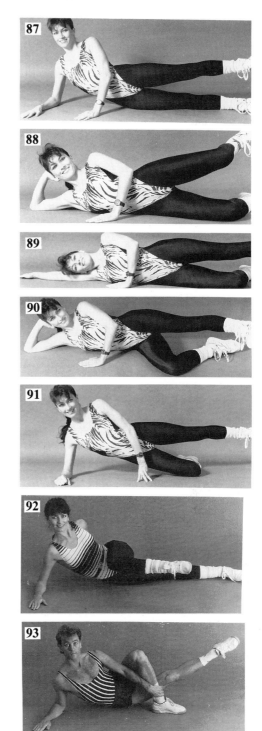

the thigh inwards as this can result in the hip flexor becoming the prime mover.

• Flex the foot and keep this horizontal. If the foot points even slightly up the hip flexors are brought more into action.

Variations:

• **Adductor raise,** (fig. 94). Lie on the side and bend the top leg so that the heel is close to the knee of the bottom leg. The bottom leg is bent and with the toes pointing slightly to the floor. Raise and lower the leg about 30 cms.

• To add further resistance straighten the lower leg (fig. 95). As a further variation raise the hips off the ground as shown in fig. 96.

• **Loaded adductor raise,** (fig. 97). This is an advanced exercise that will fatigue the adductor muscles very quickly. The body position is the same as for fig. 95 except the foot of the top leg is rested on the thigh of the lower leg. The resistance can be increased by exerting pressure on the lower leg.

Potentially dangerous exercises

The integrity of the back is compromised if the leg is forcefully or quickly raised too high as in fig. 98. To realise just how limited the range of movement is in this area try the following experiment. Adopt a hands and knees position with one leg extended behind. Contract the stomach muscles so the back is straight and well braced. Slowly raise the leg as high as possible BUT keep the back flat and allow no arch at all in the lower back. The leg cannot be raised very high. Compare this to how high some participants and instructors kick their leg in class. How do they kick the leg higher than it can be lifted? Simple, by hyperextending the lower back. A sensible, true range of motion is just as effective and more importantly, safe.

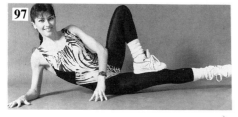

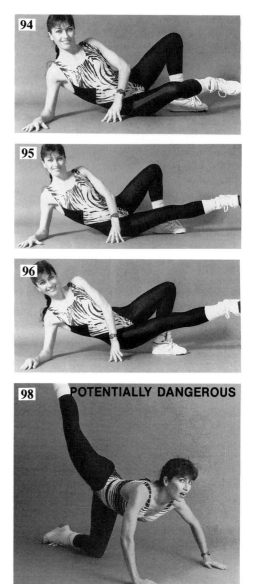

2.5 Aerobic Moves

The following are movements which can be used in an aerobics class. These can be carried out singly, or in combination with other exercises.

Standard movement

I Squatting (fig. 99)

Uses: A non impact, mild aerobic move that strengthens the thighs, particularly the extensors of the knee.

Description: Stand with feet wider than shoulder width apart, feet slightly turned out and arms above the head. Bend the knees and pull bent arms down, then straighten.

Special considerations:

• The deeper the squat the higher the load. For a warm up or for beginners only use a quarter squat (knee joint bends to approximately 135 degrees). A half squat (100 degrees) is used for a stronger workout particularly for intermediate and advanced exercisers.

- Ensure stance is wide to allow for a good range of movement and a wide base of support.

- It is imperative that the knee joint tracks properly. The knee is designed to only flex and extend in a straight line. As a general rule the knee will bend in the same direction as the foot is pointing. For most people a good squat stance is with the feet turned out anywhere from 10 to 45 degrees, therefore the knees will bend out over the foot at the same angle.

- In females there is a tendency for the knees to roll inwards or to wobble during the squatting movement. This is mainly attributed to weak vastus medialis, (inner quad muscle) and can lead to injuries.

Variations:

- **Scissor squat** (fig. 100). Start with the arms held horizontally. As the legs bend, bring straight arms down to cross or clap in front. This can be further varied by taking the arms above the head, in front of the chest or behind the back. For beginners keep

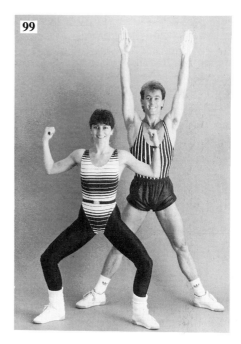

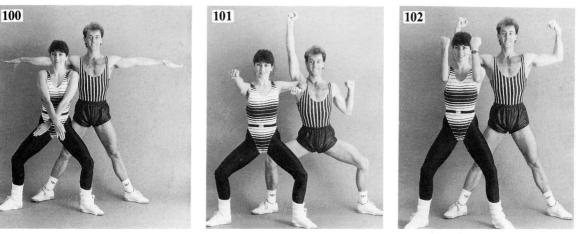

the elbows bent to shorten the lever and therefore reduce the stress on the shoulder joint. Do not pull the arms back too far or too fast and only return the arms to where they are in line with the shoulder. If pulled back further, and particularly with speed, the shoulder joint can be injured and the back hyperextended.

- **Punch squat** (fig. 101). While squatting, punch clenched fists above the head, out to the sides, in front of the body or down in front of the body. Use alternate arms or punch both out together.

- **Fly squat** (fig. 102). Start with the arms bent at 90 degrees and the upper arm horizontal. As the legs bend, pull the forearms as close to each other as possible.

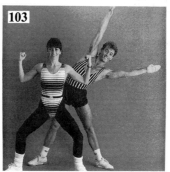

- **Reaching squat** (fig. 103). From a bent leg, bent arm position, straighten the legs and reach the extending arms out to one side. Repeat to the other side. DO NOT excessively bend the trunk to the side.

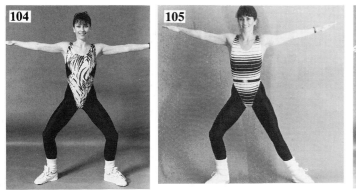

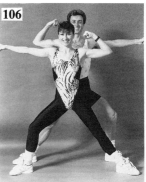

• **Hold squat** (fig. 104). Any of the above arm combinations can be performed while either holding a squat isometrically or squatting in a small range of movement without straightening the legs. This keeps a constant load on the thighs.

II Lunges (fig. 105)

Uses: A non impact, mild aerobic move that strengthens the thighs—particuarly the knee extensors and the adductors.

Description: Stand with the feet wider than shoulder width apart and turned out. Bend one knee over the foot while keeping the other leg straight.

Special considerations:
• As in the squat it is vital the knee bends in a straight line in relation to the foot. If the feet are not turned out, the knee cannot bend out therefore inhibiting the side to side movement of a lunge.

Variations:
• Add a variety of arm movements to the lunge. Some examples are reaching or punching the arms alternately or together and either up, out to the sides, across in front of the chest or down in front or behind the hips. This can be carried out with straight arms, bent arms or moving from bent to straight arms.
• **Windscreen-wiper** (fig. 106). Start with both arms horizontal as in fig. 105. When lunging to one side, bend one or both arms at the elbows. Once again this can be done above, below or in front of the body.
• **Lunge and reach** (fig. 107). While lunging to the side, stretch one arm out to the side and present the palms alternately to the ceiling. The arm movement is similar to that of throwing a frisbee.
• **Single side lunge.** Instead of lunging to alternate sides, repeat the lunge to one side with any of the arm combinations.

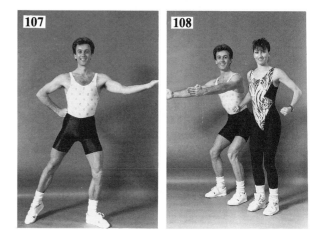

• **Lunge and swing.** While lunging to the side, swing the arms down and up in a wide circle. This can be done with single arms, both arms, or alternate arms and lunging to alternate sides.
• **Lunge and step** (fig. 108). This is stationary LIA move. Begin by bending the knees and have the arms bent and pushed back. Now step to the side and extend the arms forward. Bring the feet together and repeat on the other side.

Squatting and Lunging Combinations

Any two similar movements can be added to form combination movements. For example, repeat a squat movement for 16 counts followed by a lunge movement using the same arm action. Once the class know the two variations repeat the moves only for eight counts then four counts. This means the same movement can be repeated many times. The same principle can also be applied to other combinations e.g. repeat two different arms movements with the same squat or lunge movement, or use the same arm movement with a combination of dynamic squat or lunge.

Potential Dangers with Squats and Lunges

The knee is a hinge joint and like a door it is designed to open and close, but not to rotate or bend sideways. It is an unstable joint with much moving weight being balanced above it. To maintain integrity the joint has a complex network of ligaments, tendons and muscles whose job is to keep the knee working in its linear range of movement and to resist lateral or rotational forces. It is therefore not only potentially dangerous, but also unnatural to force the knees into rotation or side ways movements. A typical example of this is a 'skier's movement' where the knees are bent and then forced in circles. This can not only cause direct injury, but can stretch ligaments in the joint, thereby predisposing the knee to injury.

III Jumping Movements

Standard exercise:

Astride lateral jumps (fig. 109)
Uses: A moderate intensity aerobic move with emphasis on the thighs and lower leg.
Description: Start with feet together and hands by the side. Jump the feet to shoulder width apart while raising arms to the side. Flex at the ankle and knee joint upon landing to absorb the impact. Beginners use bent arms, straight arms for the more advanced.

Special considerations:
• Do not spread the legs too wide when jumping. This can stress the knee joint and cause pelvic floor and uterine ligament problems in women.
• Be cautious in swinging straight arms in a full arch from the sides to above the head. If this is done, allow more time for each movement and do not keep the hands facing out as this may stress the shoulder joint. Turn palms to the front or inward, hence relaxing the shoulders.

Variations:
• Arm variations that can be used with astride jumps are numerous. Straight arms can be scissored down in front of the body, out across the front of the chest, up above the head or down behind the back. Alternatively, the arms can be kept bent and taken through any of these directions or punched either together or alternately.
• **Opposite arm and leg,** (fig. 110). Start with the feet apart and the arms either out to the side or above the head. Pull the right elbow down and across to touch the opposite knee. This can be varied by touching the foot with the hand. A further variation is to touch one foot behind the back with the opposite hand.

Modified squat jumps (fig. 111)
Uses: A compound exercise that quickly elevates the heart rate. Emphasis is on the thighs, buttocks and lower back.

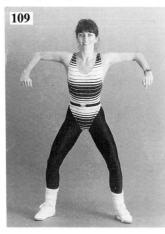

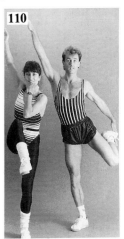

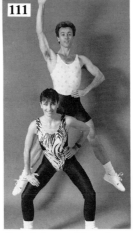

Description: Stand with the feet comfortably apart, knees bent to a quarter squat. Jump high and reach with one hand. On landing, absorb the impact in the ankles and knees by landing softly.

Special considerations:
• Do not bend the knees to a point beyond where the femur is not parallel to the floor.
• Do not touch the ground with the hands.
• On the downward phase place the hand of the outstretched arm on the thigh.

Variations:
• While jumping bring the legs together, then separate to land.
• Reach up with both arms when jumping. On landing, bring the hands down to the knees for support. This can be further varied by pushing one arm up and the other out.

Shuffle Jumps (fig. 112)

Uses: A moderate intensity aerobic move with the emphasis on the thighs and the lower leg.

Description: One leg moves jumps forward while the other is taken back. The front leg should be bent while the back leg is kept almost straight.

Special considerations:
• The heels of both feet should be grounded on landing.

Variations:
• The shuffle jump can be executed with the hands on the hips, or arm movements can be added to increase the energy cost. Figure 112 shows the arms being punched to the front. This can be done underhand or overhand.
• Punch overhead, using the opposite arm to the forward leg. This can be further varied by punching both arms out or up.
• **Arm-leg shuffle.** As the leg comes forward the same arm comes down to touch the hand to the thigh. Raise the other arm to approximately 45 degrees. Do not raise the arm too high as the music is often too fast for this long lever to travel so far.
• Clap the hands in front of the chest then pull bent elbows back and out while shuffling.
• Raise the arms laterally while shuffling.

Jump and heel touch (fig. 113)

Uses: To incorporate the front of the lower leg (anterior tibialis) into aerobic exercises. It is believed this can help reduce the incidence of lower leg injuries by strengthening the front of the leg.

Description: Start with the feet together. Move one leg to the front to touch the heel to the floor while lifting the toe (dorsi flexion). Return to the feet together position and alternate legs.

Special considerations:
• Ensure the heels are grounded and the knees stay bent.

Variations:
• Complete the shuffle without returning to the feet together position.
• Ground the heel to the side instead of the front.
• Add arm movements to any of the jump and touch movements. Curl the arms alternately or together. Punch alternate arms in any direction. Scissor the arms, bend and straighten at the elbows like windscreen-wipers, or simply reach up, out or in front of the body.

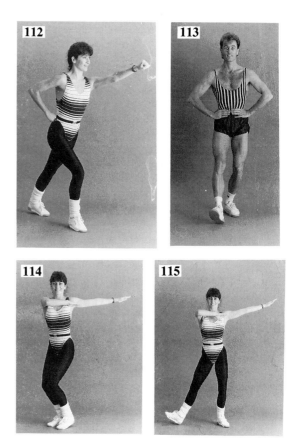

Twist jumps (fig. 114)

Uses: A moderate intensity aerobic move that incorporates the muscles of the trunk.

Description: Jump with the feet together so the hips and legs rotate to one side and the trunk and arms to the other. Reverse the movement and repeat.

Special considerations:
• As in all jumps, ground the heels on landing and keep the knees flexed.
• Do not exaggerate the twist as this could lead to back strain.
• Face forward during the movement. The arms should move across the chest and the feet and hips should turn to approximately 45 degrees in the opposite direction.

Variations:
• **Double twist.** Twist to one side, then jump in that same position before twisting to the other.
• Vary the arm position by swinging the arms down in front or over the head while twisting. It should be noted that the arm movement is similar to a

windscreen-wiper in that the elbow flexes and straightens. If the arms are kept straight, especially in the overhead position, the lever will be too long to match the speed of the leg movements.

• **Twist and touch** (fig. 114). This is similar to the standard twist, except that in twisting to one side, the outside foot should be taken further out and the heel touched to the floor. If the foot is dorsi-flexed, the tibialis anterior is brought into play.

• **Wide stance twist** (fig. 115). Twist with the feet apart in a wide stance. Perform any of the above twists with the feet shoulder width apart.

• **Rock and roll.** While performing any of the above twists, bend lower at the knees for two or four twists then straighten up for the same number.

IV Kicking (fig. 116)

Uses: Moderate intensity aerobic exercise for the legs and hip flexors.

Description: Jump on one foot while kicking the other leg to the front. Return the feet together and repeat to the other side. The opposite arm swings forward and the same arm swings back as each leg is lifted.

Special considerations:
• In most situations the leg need only be lifted to approximately 45 degrees. Too much emphasis is often placed on kicking the leg as high as possible. But this can create a ballistic effect leading to hamstring strain.

• Avoid the tendency not to ground the bottom foot properly while kicking. The bottom leg must stay slightly flexed and the heel kept on the floor. The back should be upright and the head facing forward.

Variations:
• **High kicks** (fig. 117). A high intensity kick may be suitable for intermediate to advanced exercisers. This is executed similarly to the standard kick, except that the straight leg is raised to 90 degrees. If this is difficult, keep the leg lower and avoid the tendency to sacrifice posture and form for height.

• **Flick kicks.** These are similar to the standard kick, except that the feet do not come together between kicks. As one leg is lowered, the other is prepared for the next kick by bending at the knee. Hop once on the grounded foot while the knee is brought forward and the leg flicked straight. The flick kick can also be performed to the side.

• **Bent leg kick.** This is performed in a similar fashion to the standard kick, except that the leg is

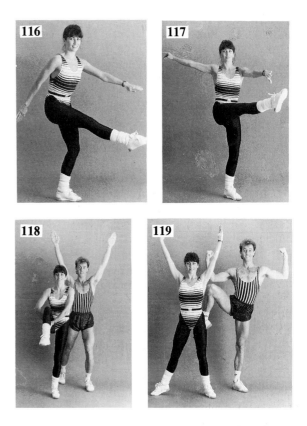

bent at the knee as it is lifted. This shortens the lever making it slightly easier but also safer.

• **Clap and kick** (fig. 118). As a bent or straight leg is kicked forward, clap the hands underneath the thigh. Beginners can clap above the thigh.

• **Side kick** (fig. 119). Raise a bent leg to the side. This can be done with the hands on the hips or made more compound by using arms movements. The arms can be pulled down from overhead as in figure 119 or clap the hands underneath the thigh as in figure 118.

• **Flutter kicks.** This involves a small, straight leg kick to the front or side. The leg is only raised 15 to 30 degrees. As one leg returns to the floor, the other is simultaneously lifted. Arms movements can also be added but will usually be limited to short lever moves such as arm curls, as the flutter kick is usually performed at a fast tempo.

• **Side swing.** Swing a straight leg out to the side while hopping on the supporting leg. Alternate legs.

V. Low Impact Aerobic (L.I.A.) Moves

Uses: For reduction of impact injuries caused by excessive jumping, running etc.

Description: These moves can range in intensity from low to high, depending on the move and the effort and range of motion involved. Low impact moves can be added to make a complete track or even an entire class. More commonly, they are used between the traditional aerobic moves. For every high impact aerobic move, there is a low impact version, and in many instances the exercise effort can be much the same. By performing an impact move, then following it with its low impact version, lower leg injuries can be reduced without reducing the overall training effect. For example, traditional lateral jumps can be performed with the arms being raised to the side. Repeat this e.g. for eight times, then perform its low impact counterpart to the right the same number of times. Repeat the standard jump eight times then the low impact version to the left eight times. This helps to make an interesting series of moves out of one simple jump. Apply the technique to any jump and the number of moves which can be used can be doubled, while instantly choreographing simple routines.

Special considerations:
• When both feet are lifted off the ground, the impact transmitted to the lower leg on landing is high. The basic principle of a low or light impact move is to reduce the impact caused in jumps, kicks and runs by keeping one foot on the ground at all times. In many instances this will also reduce the intensity of the exercises, but this can often be partially counterbalanced by keeping the supporting leg bent.

• Excessive bending of the knee of the supporting leg and forward trunk flexion have been used to maintain a high work load. But this may lead to a different range of injuries than is caused in high impact exercise. The back should normally be kept vertical and if a move requires forward flexion 10 to 15 degrees is usually enough, yet even this should not be maintained for long periods.

LIA stationary variations:
• **L.I.A. astride jump** (fig. 120). All astride jump variations can be modified. Use any arm movement, but keep one foot on the floor. The supporting leg should be slightly bent. The other leg is stepped out to the side to touch the floor. The wider the step, the higher the intensity. The move can be repeated to the one side or step to alternate sides.

• **LIA heel push** (fig. 121) Keep the supporting leg bent and push the heel of the opposite leg forward and to the floor. At the same time that the leg is being taken forward curl the opposite arm.

• **L.I.A. shuffle jump** (fig. 122). Keep the supporting

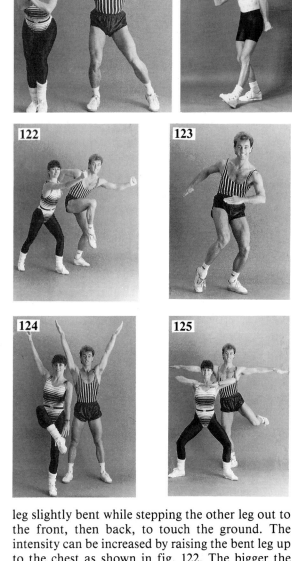

leg slightly bent while stepping the other leg out to the front, then back, to touch the ground. The intensity can be increased by raising the bent leg up to the chest as shown in fig. 122. The bigger the movement and the more effort applied, the greater the energy cost. Modify any of the combinations used for shuffle jumps.

• **L.I.A. jump and touch.** Perform the same as the impact version but do not lift both feet off the ground together. As the heel is touched out to the front or the side, keep the supporting leg underneath the body and slightly flexed.

• **L.I.A. twists** (fig. 123). Twist the body while keeping one or both feet on the ground. Twist from side to side, or lift one foot off the ground. Lift alternate arms up and down in front of the body.

- **L.I.A. kicks** (fig. 124). All the normal kicking movements can be used. Kick either a bent or straight leg to the front or side of the body. Touch one foot to the front as in fig. 124 or kick behind. Clap the hands underneath the leg or reach in the air while flicking the leg forward. Use the imagination but keep one foot on the ground.

- **L.I.A. squats** (fig. 125). Increase the intensity of the normal squat by raising one leg while returning to the upright position. Use any arm combination while lifting the leg either to the front, side or the back.

- **Step back** (fig. 126). Start with the feet together and arms by the side. Step the leg back either directly behind or to the diagonal. Combine this with an arm movement for variety.

- **Bow and arrow** (fig. 127). As one leg is stepped back, pull the arm of the same side back, while keeping the other extended. The movement is similar to drawing back on a bow. Repeat to the same side or alternate sides.

- **LIA leg flicks** (fig. 128). Begin by taking one leg back and flexing it at the knee. Both arms should be by the side of the body. Flick the leg forward while bringing the opposite arm forward. Return to the start position and repeat for the other side.

- **LIA side flicks** (fig. 129). Start the movement with the arms crossed on the chest and with one leg bent, place the ankle behind the calf of the supporting leg. Flick the bent leg to the side and extend the arms. Repeat the movement with the other leg.

- **LIA knee lifts** (fig. 130). With the hands at the sides clench the fists. Curl both arms while lifting one leg so that the thigh is parallel to the floor. Alternate legs but maintain the same arm action.

- **LIA heel touch to side** (fig. 131). Start the movement by bending the supporting leg and extending the other leg so the heel is touching the floor. Repeat the same foot pattern for the other side. Bring the arms into the movement by extending one arm and bending the other.

- **LIA step cross** (fig. 132). Start the movement with the legs apart and the arms extended out to the sides. Bring one foot across and touch the heel in front of the other leg. At the same time bend the arms and bring the elbows towards the hips. A slight variation is to have the arms above the head (fig. 133) and lower them with the step cross leg movement.

- **LIA step behind** (fig. 134). This movement is a variation to figure 132. Instead of the heel being placed in front of the supporting leg the toe touches the floor behind the supporting leg. The arm movements are the same.

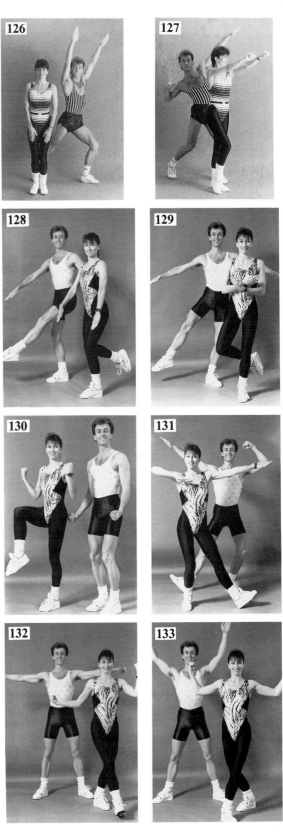

• **LIA elbow to knee** (fig. 135). This is very similar to the exercise described in figure 124. The main difference being that the elbow is brought to the opposite knee.

• **LIA step and touch** (fig. 136). Start with the legs shoulder width apart and the arms extended out to the front. Bring one leg towards the other and lower the arms so the elbows are bent and close to the hips. Repeat the movement by extending the other leg outwards and then returning it to the middle.

LIA travelling variations

In order to increase energy expenditure all travelling moves should be combined with different arm movements. However, it is important when dealing with beginners or people with poor co-ordination to teach the travelling pattern first and then introduce the arms. Also, as a rule all travelling moves should be done to four or eight counts.

• **LIA travelling: step and touch** (fig. 137). Start the travelling move by stepping out laterally and transfer the body weight onto this leg. Bring the other leg to the centre so the feet are together and repeat the move laterally.

• **LIA travelling: grapevine** (fig. 138). This travelling move is basically the same as in figure 137. But, here the travelling is done by crossing the leg behind the supporting leg. Or, as shown in figure 139 the travelling is done by crossing the leg in front of the supporting leg.

• **LIA travelling: 1,2,3 reach** (fig. 140(1)). Start the travelling move by walking forward for three counts (large steps). On the fourth count flex the hip of one leg and reach up high with the arms. Repeat the move backwards. As co-ordination improves incorporate alternate arm curls for the first three walking counts.

• **LIA travelling: 1,2,3 heel touch** (fig. 140(2)). Start the travelling move by walking forwards for three counts (large steps). On the fourth count bend the supporting leg and press the heel of the forward leg into the floor. Repeat the move backwards. As co-ordination improves incorporate arm movements such as curls, upward raises etc.

• **LIA travelling: 1,2,3 hop and turn** (fig. 141). Start the travelling move by walking fowards for three counts (large steps). On the fourth count hop and turn (on the same spot) with a high knee lift and walk for three counts back to where the travelling move commenced.

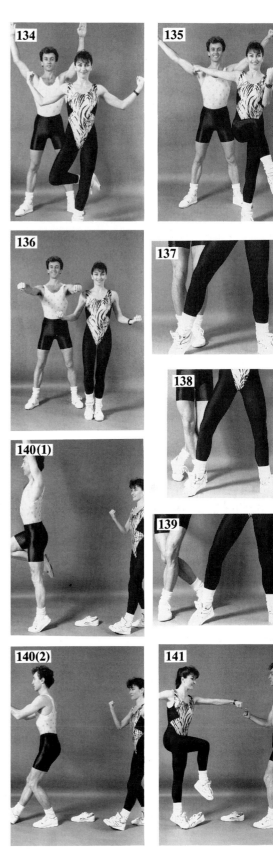

VI Running

Uses: A moderate to high intensity aerobic move.

Description: As one leg is raised, the opposite arm should also be raised and the other arm lowered. The leg is flexed at the hip and the knee. As the foot returns towards the ground, the opposite leg is lifted. The style of running in an aerobics class may be different to normal jogging, as space is limited. Most running therefore, is done on the spot.

Special considerations:
• The heel of the supporting leg must be grounded and the knee slightly flexed. Make sure the knee comes up and forward, while the heel flicks towards the buttocks.

Variations:
• **Reaching** (fig. 142). Reach the arms above the head while running. The hands can be kept open, clenched or flexed. The arms can also be pushed to the side, down or out in front.

• **Alternate punching** (fig. 143). The arms can be punched with a clenched fist either up, out, to the front or down.

• **Arm flexion running** (fig. 144). Keep the elbows high, with the upper arms horizontal. Extend and flex at the elbow. The forearm can swing out and across the chest, up and out like a windscreen-wiper, or down and out like a pendulum. The arms can move out and in together or in opposite directions.

• **Running with arm scissors.** Keep the arms straight and move these in a scissor movement to the front of the chest, above the head or below the waist. If the arms cross for every step, the movement should be small. To take the arms through a full 90 degrees in the scissor, the movement must be slowed and performed with every two steps. For added variety, start scissoring with the arms down and criss-cross the arms through an arc until they are above the head. This is usually done in four or eight steps.

• **Knees up running.** This is a high intensity move where the knees are raised as high to the front as possible. This can be performed with the hands held in front of the waist while trying to touch these with the knees.

• **Knees out running.** This is similar to the standard run, except that the knees are lifted to the side instead of to the front.

• **Heels up running** (fig. 145). Kick the heels towards the buttocks while running. In this position, the knee will not lift forward. This style of run should not be used excessively as it involves a lot of forefoot impact. Use this style only for variety. Use

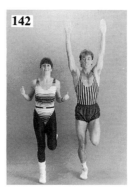
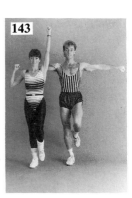
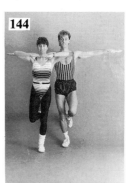
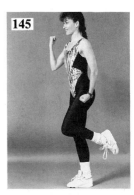
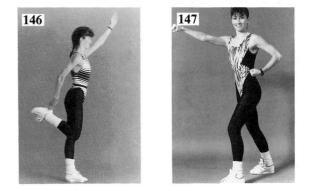

normal running arms or touch the feet with the hand as the feet kick back as shown in figure 146.

• **L.I.A. running** (fig. 147). Keep one foot on the ground and the supporting leg bent. Avoid excessive forward flexion. The arms must be pumped strongly to enhance the aerobic effect.

• **Running around the room.** If there is limited space, the normal heel-strike style associated with jogging is not possible in an aerobics class. Even with travel, landing will normally occur on the forefoot. The more limited the space the higher the knees should be raised. The larger the space the longer the step. Shorten the steps for tight corners and lengthen for the straight runs. Always counter act lateral stresses by running an equal amount in the opposite direction.

• **Race walking** (fig. 148). This is an ideal L.I.A. alternative to a travelling run. Simply walk as fast as possible around the room. Combine with an arm movement to increase the workload.

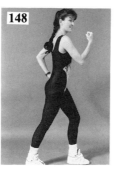

• **Isometrics** (fig. 151). The hands of one partner should be inside those of the other. While one pushes outward, the other pushes in. Stand in a squat or lunge to keep the workload high. Use the same principle for different arm positions.

• **Kicks** (figs 152 and 153). Most bent leg kicks can be performed either with partners facing as in fig. 152, or by forming lines of two or more people as in fig. 153.

• **Sit-ups** (fig. 154). With partners facing each other, sit up and clap hands in a variety of different

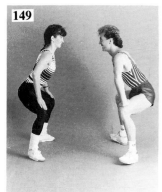

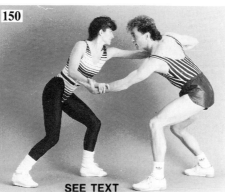

SEE TEXT

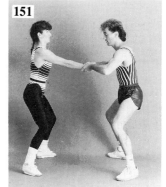

VII Partner Work

Uses: Exercising with a partner adds to the social interaction in a class and can add variety to even the most basic moves.

Special considerations:
• Although many individuals like to exercise in groups, it should be recognised that some may feel embarrassed. Participants should only be asked to touch in a class if there is a purpose. Holding hands for no apparent reason can be a turn off, not a turn on, for many people.

Variations:
• **Squatting** (fig. 149). Perform a squat facing a partner. As the legs straighten, reach out with one or both hands and clap the partner's hands. When squatting, slap the hands on the thighs. The hands can clap in front, above or to the side of the body.

• **Lunge and row** (fig. 150). Partners face each other with the same leg forward and both knees bent. Grasp the wrists and push with one arm while pulling with the other. The faster the action, the greater the effort. Please note that the pairing of partners is important as there is a strength component in this exercise that may make one partner feel uncomfortable. Also, if there is a height difference one partner may be placed in an uncompromising forward flexed position.

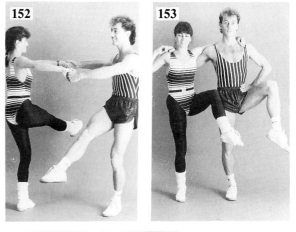

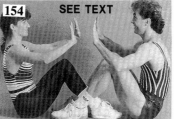

SEE TEXT

positions. Please note that when the upper body is raised more than 45 degrees off the ground the hip flexors play a primary role. For more specific abdominal work see section 2.2 of this chapter, 'Exercises for the Abdominals'.

Part B: Resistance Training Exercises

Background

Increases in technology since the industrial revolution have meant a decrease in physical exertion required in day-to-day life and an accompanying increase in obesity in Western cultures. This led to the boom in jogging in the 1970s as a means of keeping weight down and conditioning the heart and lungs. Heart disease rates, which had been climbing steadily to the mid-1970s began to decline.

In the 1980s, interest turned to body aesthetics. Those 'aerobes' of the 1970s began to appreciate that a decline in upper-body physique, accompanying activities such as jogging, was not necessarily desirable. The 'culture of narcissism', as much as anything else, has inspired a resistance revival reflected in the current boom in body building for both males and females.

But resistance training need not be aimed just at the perfect body. It can also be used as a short cut to strength, power and aerobic conditioning if carried out using the correct protocol.

1.1 Forms of Resistance

Resistance training involves any form of exercise where weight is used to increase the intensity of the exercise. This can include such things as:

- callisthenics
- barbells/dumbells
- machine systems (Universal, Nautilus, Hydragym etc.)
- aquarobics
- pulleys, levers, straps etc.

Because resistance training has been around for so long, it is unlikely that there will be many new resistance exercises discovered. Although obviously not exclusive, the exercises listed in this chapter cover all the main varieties that are used in the standard resistance training program.

There are however, new forms of resistance and new ways of carrying out all these basic exercises. Hence, while the types of exercises may not have changed, the ways of putting these together certainly have.

1.2 Uses of Resistance Training

Resistance can be used for one or more of the following 4 purposes:

- to increase strength
- to improve power
- to add to body bulk, or
- to develop aerobic conditioning.

Strength is the ability to exert force

Power is the ability to exert force in a short period of time

Bulking refers to hypertrophy of muscle tissue to increase size

Aerobic conditioning is the capacity of the heart and lungs to pump blood to the working muscles.

1.3 Training Regimes

Resistance training regimes will vary according to the requirements of the program. Variations in general are based on:

1. Repetitions (reps), or the number of times an exercise is repeated. In general the higher the repetitions the more the emphasis is on aerobic conditioning.

2. Sets, or the number of groups of repetitions of an exercise. Ideally it is thought that 3–5 sets of an exercise is ideal. But for maximum overload, this may be increased up to 15.

3. Resistance, or the amount of weight used. Heavy weights are used for strength and power development, medium/heavy weights for bulk,

and light/medium weights for aerobic conditioning. Individual weights are determined by the concept of *Repetition Maximum* (RM), which is the maximum number of repetitions which can be carried out with a single weight (e.g. 10 RMs would be the weight that an individual could lift 10 times only).

4. Rest is necessary for the regrowth of muscle tissue after overload. Generally, it is thought that rest is required over a 24 hour period for muscle groups involved in resistance training.

The table summarises the types of regimes to be carried out for the various benefits from resistance training. In certain circumstances a combination of these can be carried out i.e. for aerobic conditioning and bulk.

Resistance Training Regimes

Purpose	Weight	Repetitions	Sets	Exercise Speed	Rest between sets
Strength	Very heavy (90%–100% RM)	2– 6	3– 5	Slow/medium	30 secs–2 mins
Power	Heavy (80%–90% RM)	2– 6	3– 5	Fast	30 secs–2 mins
Body bulk	Heavy (70%–90% RM)	6–12	3–10	Slow	Unlimited
Aerobic conditioning	Light/medium (40%–60% RM)	12–30	*	Fast	Minimal

*Sets are not important here. It is the number of exercises that counts.

1.4 Forms of Muscle Training

There are 3 main types of muscle contraction of interest to the weight trainer:

1. Isometric training:
The term isometric comes from the Greek *isos metrikos* meaning literally 'the same length' or 'no change in length'. Isometric (or static) exercises are those where a muscle develops tension without changing length. In fact, the muscle does shorten internally during an isometric contraction, but this is countered by a contraction of the antagonist muscle or the resistance of an immovable object.

Isometric training originated in the early 1950s after 2 German scientists, Hettinger and Muller

reported a 5% increase in strength following daily isometric exercises. The exercises were carried out with a tension of two-thirds of maximum strength held for 6 seconds at a time.

In the 1960s isometrics became popular amongst sedentary workers who were unable to get out for more active involvement. In the 1970s it was reported to be of limited value, particularly in the absence of an aerobic routine: more so, it was often thought to be dangerous, particularly for those with a weak heart. This is because it was thought that isometrics have a greater effect on blood pressure than exercises that involve muscle shortening.

Now, isometrics is again thought to have value *in certain circumstances* and even in cases of cardiac rehabilitation. Research is continuing to determine the most effective training regimes.

Some of the best improvements have been measured in programs using 5–10 contractions at maximal strength held for 5 seconds each. These have come from programs carried out over 3 days a week, but the optimal training frequency is considered to be 5 days a week. Training can be combined with isotonic work-outs.

Isometrics are useful for developing strength in weak spots and for increasing strength and preventing injury at the limits of the range of motion. However, it should be recognised that they only build strength at the specific angle at which they are carried out. Hence to develop total muscle power, an isometric force should be applied at 4 or 5 different angles in the joint range of motion.

Isometrics are particularly useful for sports such as judo, gymnastics and windsurfing, where a position may have to be held for some time.

2. Isotonic training:

The term isotonic literally means 'of equal tension'. It implies that the muscle develops a certain tension or force in lifting a load. In fact, the force developed by the muscle is variable depending on the joint angle and the efficiency of the lever at that joint.

An isotonic (dynamic) contraction, is one in which muscular force is developed in lifting a constant resistance throughout the range of motion of the joint. Isotonic training with weights was developed in the late 1940s using the concept of *Repetition Maximums* (RM) for determining the amount of weight used. An RM is defined as the maximal load a muscle or muscle group can lift a given number of times before fatiguing.

For years it has been thought that strength could be improved only by using heavy resistance with low repetitions, and endurance by using light resistance with high repetitions. Recent studies have shown however, that there is a good deal of carry-over from one type of training to another, even though the basic principle may still apply.

3. Isokinetic training:

An isokinetic contraction is one in which maximal tension is developed throughout the full range of movement. This requires special equipment in which the speed of the movement is kept constant over the full range of movement regardless of the tension applied. Hence if the movement is made as fast as possible, the tension generated by the muscles will be maximal throughout the full range of motion.

Isokinetic training is relatively new and has therefore not yet been extensively evaluated scientifically. Research that has been carried out has shown significant strength gains. But in comparison with other isotonic devices the gains are relative to the type of equipment used for evaluation. For example, athletes trained on isokinetic machines develop greater increases in strength than athletes trained isotonically, *if the measure of strength is isokinetic*. If the measure is isotonic, the opposite is true.

Isokinetic training is particularly useful in the rehabilitation of injury and in sports training which requires maximal power output throughout the full range of a muscle contraction. Furthermore, because isokinetic contractions can be made at speed, this type of training can assist in power and speed for various sporting activities.

1.5 Resistance Programming

The following are the steps involved in resistance programming:

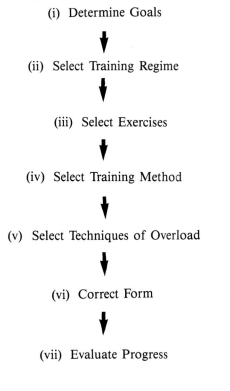

(i) Determine Goals

(ii) Select Training Regime

(iii) Select Exercises

(iv) Select Training Method

(v) Select Techniques of Overload

(vi) Correct Form

(vii) Evaluate Progress

1.6 Classifying Strength-Training Methods

One problem in resistance training has always been in classifying methods. Many taxonomies exist, but these are often confusing. Perhaps one of the clearest is a recent attempt by German sport scientist Dr Dietmar Schmidtbleicher.

Schmidtbleicher categorises weight-training methods into 4 major groups based on intensity of muscle contractions. The groups are:

- Maximum Strength (Contractions) Methods
- Submaximal Contraction Methods
- Reactive Methods
- Strength-Endurance Methods

An explanation of each, its various sub-categories and main benefits is summarised below.

(a) Maximal strength methods

These are used for maximal strength development (with minimal bulking). They involve contractions against heavy loads (i.e. 90–100% RM) or supra-maximal loads (150% +) and can be expected to produce effects within 6–8 weeks with 4 training units per week. Main effects come from improvements in neural co-ordination. Techniques include:

1. Near maximal concentric contractions:
May be 3–4 sets with weight increasing from 90% RM to 100% in the last set.

2. Maximal concentric contractions:
Should be used only by experienced strength athletes (e.g. power lifters, etc. uses 4–5 sets of 1 rep at 100% load with a 3–5 minute rest).

3. Maximal isometric contractions:
Mainly used in rehabilitation or for isometric strength sports. Weight is 100% and 1–2 isometric contractions (no movement) are carried out for 4–5 sets. Rest should be 3 minutes.

4. Maximal eccentric contractions:
(Also called 'negative reps'). Load can be up to 150% RM and spotters are needed such that weight is only lowered. Three sets of 4–5 reps are carried out with 3 minute rests. Again, to be used only by experienced strength athletes.

5. Concentric-eccentric maximal contractions:
The eccentric phase in this form is exaggerated to cause a deceleration in the lowering phase, while the upward (concentric) phase is accelerated [i.e. 2 seconds concentric (upward), and 4 seconds eccentric (downward)]. Uses 3–5 sets of 6–8 reps with 70–90% RM weight. Often used by power-strength athletes.

(b) Sub-maximal contraction repetition methods

These methods use submaximal loads (60–80%) over a large number of reps to failure. Results are increases in muscle mass within 10–12 weeks of 4 sessions per week. The technique, unlike A, is not totally effective for strength or explosive sports, but may be used for endurance sports and bulking. Techniques include:

1. Standard method I:
With load of 80%, 3–5 sets of 8–10 reps. Probably the most common technique used, particularly for beginners.

2. Standard method II:
As with (i) but with a progressively increasing load i.e. 12 reps with 70% down to 5 reps at 90% over 4–5 sets. Final set should be carried out to failure. Better for advanced bulk training.

3. Pyramiding method:
Many varieties are used but generally begins with light weight working up to heavy by adding weight and decreasing reps in each set then decreasing weight to failure. Rest of 2–3 minutes between sets.

4. Body-building method I:
Aims to completely fail muscles. Load is 60–70% and 3–5 sets of 15–20 reps are carried out with a rest of 2–3 minutes. Results in increased blood flow and capillarisation of muscle and therefore bulk.

5. Body-building method II:
Seeks a more intensive failure of muscle by 2–5 sets of 5–8 reps at 85–95% RM.

Within the 2 body-building techniques are a number of variations including:

- **Forced reps:** Where assistance is given to achieve greater failure at the end of a set.
- **Negative reps:** Eccentric contractions carried out with assistance at the end of a normal set.

- **Supersets:** Two sets of complementary exercises with no rest between.
- **'Burning' reps:** Incomplete reps at the end of a set of 6 RM. 'Burning' sensation comes from (unsuccessful) attempts to complete the range of motion.
- **Cheating reps:** Completing reps by bringing in an assisting muscle group (e.g. bending the back in as in arm curls).
- **Pre-exhaustion:** Isolating a muscle in one set, then exhausting to failure by following with a compound exercise (see below).

6. Isokinetic training:
Can only be carried out with special equipment which provides accommodating resistance for every joint angle, hence producing a constant speed of contraction. Thought to be useful where sports involve isokinetic resistance (e.g. swimming, rowing).

7. Isometric method:
Generally used in rehabilitation. Maximum contractions of from 1–12 reps for 3–5 sets. Also used in sports where some isometric contractions are involved (e.g. martial arts, skiing, windsurfing etc).

8. Speed-strength method:
With light load (35–50% RM) over 7 reps carried out with rapid speed in the concentric phase. Useful for light power sports e.g. javelin.

(c) Strength-endurance methods

These involve developing strength over a length of time required for an endurance event, hence requiring a greater use of the aerobic energy system than in other methods. Techniques include:

1. Strength-endurance method I:
Uses 3–5 sets of 10–20 reps with loads of 40–60% and minimal rest.

2. Strength-endurance method II:
Slightly less intensive with 4–6 sets of 30 reps and load of 20–40% and minimal rest. Used more where aerobic benefit and/or weight loss are required.

(d) Reactive training methods
These methods involve training for speed and strength in movements that involve sudden shortening of muscles in power movements (such as jumping, or sprinting). The technique can lead to injury and must be used carefully. Techniques include:

1. Hop training:
Trying to gain maximal height with each of 30 reps. Can be done on one or both legs. May also be 3 sets of 10 reps with 5 minute rest intervals.

2. Jump training:
Alternate step-hopping for 3–4 sets of 20 reps. Can be done over 50 metres with maximum distances attempted. May also be done slowly as 'bounding'. Mainly for leg power.

3. Plyometrics:
Also called 'depth jumping'; involves jumping from height where the heel does not touch the ground and bounding up to a higher height. Can be done in 3–5 sets of 10 reps for jumpers and sprinters. Upper-body plyometrics i.e. explosively 'throwing' a weight in the bench press can be used for field events such as shot put.

1.7 Modern Techniques of Overload

Overload is the key to improvement in any form of resistance training. It simply means overloading a muscle to the point where changes have to occur structurally for the muscle to adapt to the overload.

Traditionally, overload has been supplied through increased resistance, sets or repetitions of an exercise. More esoteric overloading techniques, sometimes based on unclear physiological principles, have been used particularly by body-builders and sports trainers for years.

In fact, this is one aspect of exercise training where the practice has often preceded the theory.

It is clear also that individuality has to be taken into consideration in evaluating overloading practices. Where some individuals respond well to some overloading techniques, others do less well. Hence it is important for a fitness leader to know the range of techniques available.

The following is a list of overload techniques gathered from sports training and body-building practices.

Blitzing is the practice of bombarding a muscle or muscle group on any one training day. This can take the form of several exercises aimed at working the muscle from different angles.

Blitzing is obviously a fatiguing technique, and therefore not recommended during peaking for sports competition.

Pyramiding refers to the practice of increasing resistance step by step over sets or repetitions. It can also be combined with a reduction in repetitions over sets. For example, if an exercise is done with X weight over 10 repetitions in set 1, it may be one with X + 10% X weight over 8 repetitions in set 2, and X + 20% X weight over 6 repetitions in set 3.

Reverse pyramiding is where the weight is decreased step by step as per the pyramiding principle, to allow a greater number of repetitions to be carried out. This technique is more relevant where a muscle has been worked to fatigue, in order to squeeze more effort from that muscle.

Forced repetitions require a partner or 'spotter' such that assistance can be given in that part of the movement where biomechanical advantage is least, and hence where the muscle is weakest. This then means a heavier weight can be lifted through the full range of movement.

For example, in the arm curl motion, a 'sticking point' is reached about where the elbows are at right angles. If assistance is given through this point, a heavier weight can be used through the full range of motion.

Cheating is a technique only recommended for experienced weight trainers where an auxiliary muscle is used to assist a prime mover in a movement. For example, in arm curls the body is bent through contraction of the back muscles to enable the lifter to lift a heavier weight through the weakest point of the movement. This means a heavier weight can be used and the muscle is thus overloaded all the way through the movement.

Negative repetitions capitalise on the fact that strength and bulk improvements in muscle are aided by exaggerated eccentric (lowering) contractions of a muscle. In a negative repetition the weight is only lowered enabling more weight to be used to overstress the muscle eccentrically. Spotters are generally required to lift the weight for the lifter so that this can then be lowered.

An example of negative repetitions would be where the weight is lowered to the chest slowly in the bench press and then returned to the rack by spotters so the action can be repeated. Eccentric contractions are thought to place greater stress on muscle tissue than concentric actions because of the negative use of gravity in the former.

Pre-exhaustion is where a muscle is isolated in an exercise and fatigued before being co-opted for further work in a compound exercise which immediately follows. The second, or compound exercise, enables the muscle previously exhausted to continue working because it is aided by synergists.

Examples of pre-exhaustion are dumbell flies followed by bench press for the pectorals, lateral raises followed by military press for the deltoids and leg extensions followed by squats for the quadriceps.

Rest Pause is a technique practised by body-builders for increasing intensity of effort. It is done by overloading a muscle such that only one repetition can be carried out and a pause is necessary (perhaps 6–8 seconds), before it can be done again and again, over a set number of repetitions.

This is a high-intensity technique that should only be carried out by experienced lifters.

Up and Down the Rack is a principle similar to pyramiding, except that weights from light to heavy gradations are arranged on a weight rack and exercises carried out with each of these, and with weight increasing and then decreasing, until exhaustion.

Super-Setting is a method of combining 2 exercises without a rest period in between. The 2 exercises may be used to 'blitz' a muscle, or may in fact work agonist and antagonist muscles. It increases overload both in intensity and in potential aerobic benefit.

Giant Sets are super-sets with more than 2 exercises carried out without rest in between. This technique is more appropriate for the athlete requiring aerobic conditioning as well as strength.

Peripheral Heart Action (PHA) is a technique which brings in aerobic conditioning by exercising muscle groups some distance from each other on the body, in successive exercises. This means blood is shunted rapidly throughout the body putting more pressure on the heart and lungs, and thus increasing aerobic effort.

Peak Contractions are where a muscle is totally contracted, thus resulting in maximal contraction of all muscle fibres simultaneously. If the muscle is overloaded at this point, it is assumed that greater stimulation of more fibres will occur.

The best exercises for peak contraction are those where the lifter has to 'fight' to hold the weight at the end of the range of movement. This includes such exercises as chin-ups, leg extensions, tricep push-downs etc.

1.8 Compound and Isolation Exercises

Having selected the right regime, the next step is to select the most appropriate exercises for the task. Basically, there are 2 types:

1. Compound exercises: are those that involve more than one major muscle or muscle group. Because of the large muscle mass involved, these types of exercise use more energy and are therefore better for overall aerobic conditioning and weight-loss programs.

2. Isolation exercises: are those where a specific muscle is isolated for the purpose of strengthening or enlarging that muscle. These types of exercises generally involve little overall energy use and are more specific to strength training or body-building programs.

There are obviously many compound and isolating exercises available. However a selection of 5 of the best of each can give a variety of exercises which, in total or in some combination, can be used in any resistance training program.

1.9 Choosing the Best Equipment

Where weights are used, there is a variety of machines and training systems available. And while the manufacturers of each often claim special advantages, no one machine system caters for all contingencies. All have their advantages and disadvantages and there is even controversy over the use of free weights versus machines. For example:

For free weights

Transfer of training Specificity of training is a key aspect of strength and fitness development for sports. With free weights, it has been suggested that the individual's own pattern of motor unit firing, used in non weight training performance, can be simulated closely. This is because the freely-moving bar is not being 'guided' or otherwise restrained as would be the case with machine movement.

Joint strength Because the free weight user has to balance the resistance rather than be guided by machinery, the controlling action is suggested to be an aid in developing joint strength.

Muscle synergism Many exercise machines are constructed to isolate one or a limited number of muscles and work intensively on these. Free weights, it is argued, offer better total muscle group conditioning than machine systems, therefore offering greater economy of training.

Individuality Some machine systems are designed to provide variable resistance through the full range of movement. However, to do so, they rely on force-angle relationships which are based on estimates from the *average* person. Individual differences in limb length, point of muscle attachment, muscle architecture, velocity of movement etc., mean that certain individuals may be restricted in their movements because inappropriate workloads may be applied at various angles. This does not occur with free weights.

Psychological factors Although not proven, it has been suggested that athletes are more motivated to improve their strength performance on free weights. This is because of the greater satisfaction of improving poundage and personal best performances with loose weights.

For the machine systems

Safety Because machines systems are generally attached within a unit there are safety advantages that are not present with heavy loose weights. Some manufacturers also claim that there is less chance of injury through incorrect movements if the range of movement is fixed.

Cheating As for safety, the fixed movements of many weight systems ensure that an exercise is carried out correctly and that 'cheating' cannot occur.

Compactness There is little question that most machine systems are more compact and neat, and therefore more physically attractive in many gym situations than loose weights. They also offer the advantage that many people can be trained simultaneously.

Rehabilitation training The guided action and variable resistance of some machine systems makes them particularly suited to injury rehabilitation training. Less strain is likely to be put on injured joints than with free weights.

General fitness training Where specific muscle strength, as in sport training, is not the aim of a program, machine systems may be of more advantage than free weights. Certain systems may be of particular advantage in circuit training.

1.10 Variations in Training from Beginner to Advanced

Technique and prescription are 2 vital aspects of any weight-training program. And most standard instructional texts have set approaches to both.

Yet just as a beginner would not be given the same amount of weight to lift as an advanced exerciser, there are lifting techniques which also change with experience. Some of these are not covered in the standard texts. For example:

1. Feet positioning in the bench press: Commercially made bench-press benches are often long enough only to accommodate the torso to the base of the pelvis in the supine position.

This means the legs are left to hang over the edge of the bench. They can either be positioned flat on the floor, in which case the back is arched, or placed in the air or on the end of the bench, thus flattening the back.

An arched (and unsupported) back, is potentially dangerous for the inexperienced or those with lower back problems. Hence, the beginner should be taught either to raise the feet to an extension of the bench, or cross the legs in the air so the back is flattened. On the other hand, an experienced lifter using a heavy weight may need to keep the feet flat on the floor for extra support.

2. Use of machines versus free weights: Machine systems in resistance training have a distinct safety advantage over free weights. Because the action is guided, it is more difficult for the beginner to carry out an exercise incorrectly. It is also more appropriate for learning the correct technique for later progression to free weights.

Free weights offer advantages over machine systems however in that support muscles are used, joints are strengthened and the action is more like 'real life'.

The correct progression then would be from machine systems to free weights where the actions are duplicated.

3. Progressions in the squat: The squat is one of the best overall compound exercises available. But it has inherent dangers, particularly because of the pressure placed on knee ligaments when the knee is flexed beyond 90 degrees. Orthopaedic studies have shown that the shearing force on the knee can increase by up to 7 times that of the weight being carried when the knee is flexed beyond this position.

Other problems with the squat are:
- the difficulty in performing the exact technique such that maximum benefits are gained, and
- the tendency to cheat in order to carry a heavy load.

For the beginner, any of the standard squat machines can help develop technique. However, the beginner should never be put into the full squat position.

Often, lack of flexibility in the Achilles tendon leads to a tendency to want to place the heels on a raised block. But this only exacerbates the problem. The beginner then should be taught to squat only to a point that is comfortable with the heels on the floor and not beyond the position of thighs parallel to the floor. As flexibility improves, allowing greater movement, the squat can, with caution, be taken lower.

Other changes which can be made with advanced training include changes in feet position (toes in/out etc.), changes in the position of the bar (back of neck versus front of chest), and changes in weight used.

4. Flexed hip sit-ups: Beginners to an exercise program are generally weak in the abdominals. To compensate, the hip flexors are often over-stressed by locking the feet in a straight leg position for the sit-up.

More emphasis is put on the abdominals when the hips are flexed, and the hip flexor muscles are relaxed. But in this position many beginners cannot raise their shoulders off the ground. However, in the early stages, this is probably enough.

The superior portion of rectus abdominus is worked by raising head and shoulders off the ground in this position. With increased strength, the upper body can be raised further off the ground. Another progression with experience is to the side sit-up and twist, this time with feet locked but body turned on the side and twisted to the front during the action.

5. Increased sets/decreased reps: In the early part of a weight-training program, large increases in strength can come from one set of relatively low-resistance exercise. This has the added advantage of minimising muscle soreness and reducing the risk of injury.

Only with experience should weight be increased, ensuring correct technique. Repetitions can be decreased from 15–20 per set to 6–8 per set

and weight increased accordingly. Sets can then be increased to provide greater muscle overload once muscle groups have adapted.

6. From uniformity to periodisation: For a beginner, the most important aspect of a weight-training program is learning technique and muscle adaptation. Hence, uniformity of a training program over 3–4 days a week is important, with gradual progressions in resistance, repetitions ec.

For the more advanced exerciser on the other hand, greater advances are made from periodising exercise; that is changing the program over a set period of either weeks or months.

A regime of light weights with high repetitions can be used for 3–6 weeks, followed by a period of 3–6 weeks with heavy weights and low repetitions. This can then lead into a third cycle, where the weight is relatively light again, although at a higher level than in phase 1. Greater strength developments have been shown using this technique than the uniform training approach.

7. From 'compound' to 'isolation': Isolation exercises (i.e. those using predominantly a prime mover muscle), have little value to a beginning exerciser looking for increases in aerobic fitness as well as general improvements in muscle tone.

Energy usage in isolation work is generally lower than with compound exercises (i.e. those with more than one muscle or group involved). With improved general fitness more isolation work may be included in order to improve on specific muscle development. Hence the beginner would concentrate on compound movements, the advanced on a compound/isolation mix.

1.11 Weight Training and Weight Loss

Exercise prescription for weight control in the gymnasium setting often involves a weight training regime. Connotations of muscle tone from weight training mean that this is often the desired form of training by both programmer and client. But while extensive and regular weight training combined with rigid nutritional regulation may have good results, the value of moderate-intensity weight training alone in weight control is now coming under question.

Research on the energy costs of weight-training techniques has recently shown some surprises. The effort exerted in a typically moderate gym routine for example, may be little different from walking at a brisk pace.

In one recent co-operative study carried out by scientists at 4 U.S. universities, energy use was measured directly by oxygen consumption in 4 males familiar with weight-training techniques.

Energy was measured for exercises carried out

for (a) the chest, shoulders and arms, and (b) the back and legs using exercise machines. Each exercise was repeated 6–9 times in sets of 3 using 75–80% of maximum load which could be lifted for one repetition.

The program was standardised so that exercises were carried out in 3 × 3 second work sets separated by a 1 minute rest and followed by a 2.5 minute final rest period. This gave a total workout period of 36 minutes.

Results showed that the average energy expenditure during exercise was 6.7 kilocalories per minute for upper-body work and 8.2 kilocalories per minute for lower-body—or between 174–222 kilocalories per session. The findings have been supported by similar studies carried out by each of the scientists involved.

Given that resting energy levels are between 1–2 kilocalories per minute, and this is barely the energy expenditure of a 3 km walk, the implications for fat reduction are limited.

Implications for Exercise Programming

It is commonly thought that even moderate weight-lifting sessions expend large amounts of energy, hence explaining the low body fat and high muscle bulk of athletes and body builders.

However, it should be remembered that these individuals carry out 2–5 times the work load of that tested here—even though the lower work-load is more characteristic of that prescribed for the average weight-control client in the gym setting.

Weight training alone then, would appear to have little benefit in a weight-control program. Practices which may improve the efficiency of weight training for fat reduction include:

- decreasing rest periods between sets;
- working for longer periods with lighter weights;
- using *compound* rather than *isolation* exercises;
- programming exercise using the larger muscles of the body (thighs, trunk, shoulders);
- circuit training.

1.12 Guidelines for Resistance Training

The following are guidelines for strength and body shape training adapted from the document 'Standards and Guidelines for the Planning and Conduct of Fitness Programs' published by the Australian Fitness Accreditation Council.

1. The type of strength training will depend on the requirements of the training program. Isometric exercise for example, will be appropriate in situations where isometric strength is required. It is appropriate therefore that the exercise and equipment suit the purpose.

2. Particular attention should be paid to safety of equipment and exercises designed for the purpose. Individual counselling is advisable to assess structural weaknesses or abnormalities in clients.

3. A strength-training routine should involve the use of the 'overload' principle i.e. progressively heavier weights or an increasing number of repetitions.

4. Weight standards should be determined at the outset for each client. These can then be adjusted according to improvement.

5. All equipment used must meet the standards set down for exercise equipment by the relevant bodies.

6. Strength training should not be confused with aerobic conditioning and no suggestion should be made to a client that strength training exercises will improve aerobic fitness.

7. Individual record cards should be available for clients so that workouts can be standardised and efforts recorded. Regular monitoring of cards by an Instructor should occur and this should be accompanied by regular consultations with the client.

8. There must be no use of 'passive' exercise equipment in strength training except for the purposes of massage or relaxation, in which case the client should be advised of such purpose.

9. Adequate warm-up and cool-down provisions should apply to strength programs as to other exercise programs.

10. Stretching (static or PNF [see page 80]) should be carried out after a strength workout to relieve excessive muscle tension.

11. Heavy resistances should not be used until lifting techniques are perfected.

12. Exercise should involve opposing (agonist/antagonist) muscle groups and aim for bilateral development of these groups.

13. Caution must be taken with resistance exercises involving hyperextension of the lower back and with exercises involving extreme joint flexion.

14. Exercises should be carried out with smooth, even rhythm, moving weights through the full range of joint motion.

15. Clients should be advised that inhalation should occur on the lifting of a weight and exhalation on the lowering of that weight. Breath should not be held at any time.

16. Clients should be advised on correct techniques for lifting weights from the floor, on feet positioning during lifting of free weights where appropriate, and on the correct grip to be applied to equipment.

17. Care should be taken to ensure that children are not in the locality of heavy weights or strength training equipment and that weights are stored safely when not in use.

18. Exercises for body shaping must be of the type that will genuinely influence body shape. For example, mild callisthenics or stretching exercises are not considered to fall within this category.

19. Where weight loss is an objective, an aerobic component should be incorporated in the exercise session.

20. There should be no credence given to 'spot reduction' that does not involve general aerobic exercise with specific muscle toning.

21. There must be no use made of techniques for weight control such as figure wrapping, creams, electric stimulators or other such devices for which no sound body of credibly published scientific evidence exists.

22. Some emphasis should be given to providing nutritionally sound advice to clients regarding food intake to supplement a body shaping exercise program.

23. The use of heat treatments (sauna, swirl or steam baths) must be restricted for clients who may be overweight, suffer high blood pressure or be over 45 years of ago. Such devices should not be used for weight loss purposes with other clients and no suggestion should be made that this is their purpose.

24. Where heat treatments are used, information on their risks and benefits must be made clearly available for all clients.

25. All exercises must be carried out correctly, particularly avoiding bouncy and jerky movements. Clients using standard gymnasia equipment should be advised of the manufacturer's specifications for exercise on each piece of equipment.

26. Advice should be given to clients about the frequency, intensity and duration of effort required to achieve desired results.

27. Particular care should be given to clients with high blood pressure.

2. The Exercises

2.1 Exercises for the Arms

I. Biceps

Standard exercise

1. The barbell curl (fig. 155)
Uses: Develops the biceps and brachialis as well as the muscles of the forearm.
Description: This is the standard biceps exercise. While standing with feet shoulder-width apart and knees slightly bent, curl the arms with an under-hand grip. One leg may be placed forwards for extra stabilisation. The back should be kept straight and the upper arms by the sides. The brachialis is emphasised more if the elbows are kept into the sides.

Special considerations
• lower the weight slowly,
• do not lean back unless specifically attempting to 'cheat' the movement.

Variations
• **Cheating curl.** This is carried out by bending the back to help move through the 'sticking point' in the movement. Cheating should only be carried out by experienced lifters.

• **True biceps curl** (fig. 156), is where the elbows do not stay by the side, thus making the biceps (and not brachialis) the prime movers, and bringing in the deltoids as 'helper' or synergist muscles.

• **Easy curl bar** [*see preacher curl*]. This allows a more natural rotation of the arm in flexion and therefore offers greater protection against injury for the regular weight-trainer.

• **Wide/narrow grip curl.** Varies the emphasis on outer and inner biceps and changes the emphasis on synergists from deltoids to pectorals.

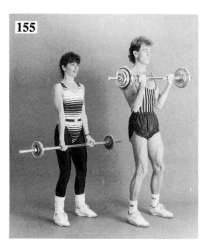

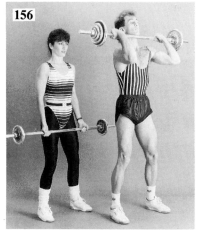

• **Seated curls,** or curling while lying prone or supine on an incline bench, kneeling down etc. are other options which can change the emphasis on the upper arm muscles.

Other exercises

2. Preacher curl (fig. 157)

Uses: Helps bulk the lower biceps and brachialis muscles and can help lengthen the muscles of the upper arm.

Description: The arms are rested over a bench and with the elbows fixed, the forearm is flexed to shoulder level. Lower the weight slowly.

Special considerations
• Ensure that the arms are taken through the full range of motion;
• Do not lean back in the lifting phase.

Variations
• **Wide/narrow grip preacher curl** (fig. 158). A wide grip works the medial portion of the biceps. The hands should be shoulder-width apart on the bar. With the grip narrowed, the emphasis is placed more on the lateral portion of the biceps.

• **Dumbell preacher curl.** Dumbells can be substituted for a barbell where one arm is stronger than the other. This prevents injuries caused by compensation of one muscle group for another.

3. Dumbell curl (fig. 159)

Uses: Stretches the biceps and allows independent development in cases where one arm may be stronger than the other.

Description: Keep the back upright and curl the forearms towards the shoulders. This can be done with the arms alternately, or both together. To maximise the contraction, twist the wrist at the top of the curl so although the palm is facing upwards, the thumb points downwards.

Variations
• **Seated or standing dumbell curls** vary the comfort level of the exercise.

• **Lying dumbell curls.** The position of the action can be changed by lying face down or face up on a bench (incline, decline or level). This helps to keep the upper body fixed, and varies the emphasis on the biceps.

• **'Hammer curl'.** Turn the palms to face inwards and keep them at this angle through the curling movement. The outer edge of the forearm is worked more in this position.

• **Dumbell clean with curl** (fig. 160). By reaching to the floor, then standing upright and curling the dumbells, the action is made a more 'compound' movement.

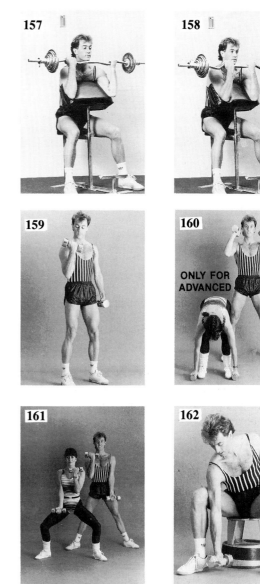

• **Dumbell curl with squat** (fig. 161). Bending the legs while curling with the dumbells means more energy is involved and thus makes the exercise useful for circuit training or aerobic conditioning.

4. Concentration curl (fig. 162)

Uses: Develops a 'peaking' of the biceps.

Description: The concentration curl makes use of gravity through the full range of motion, thereby putting greater stress on the biceps. Bend forwards from a seated or standing position and curl the forearm towards the shoulder. Lower slowly.

5. Two arm cable curl (fig. 163)

Uses: Develops and shapes the biceps and brachialis.

Description: The action is identical to the standard barbell curl. Tension is maintained through the full upward of motion because there is no gravitational effect at the top of the motion.

Variations

• **Wide/narrow grip cable curl.** Changing the grip changes the emphasis from the inner biceps (wide grip), to the outer biceps (narrow grip).

• **Preacher bench cable curl.** Using a preacher bench makes the movement more strict and less amenable to 'cheating'.

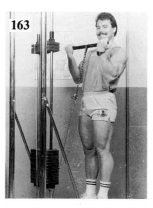

6. One arm cable curl (fig. 164)

Uses: Develops independent unilateral biceps strength.

Description: The basic action is similar to a dumbell curl except that constant tension is provided throughout the full range of motion with cables (*note:* constant tension with standard cables does not mean 'isokinetic' tension). Unilateral movement allows for strength differences between the arms which may result in injury in a two-handed action. This type of movement is good for sports where independent arm strength is required e.g. canoeing.

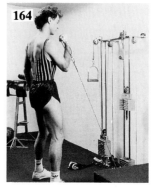

Variations

• **One arm cross-over cable curls** (fig. 165). Pull the cable across the body until the arm is fully flexed. Biceps are actively involved in this action.

• **One arm cable curls.** Use a preacher bench to create a stricter, more intense movement for advanced peaking.

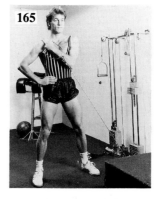

7. Reverse grip pull-down (fig. 166)

Uses: Involves the biceps in a compound action including lats and intercostal muscles.

Description: Using a lat pull-down machine, palms facing towards the body, pull down until the elbows are by the side. This can be used as a substitute for chin-ups in females because of the varied weight which can be used.

Variations

• **Wide/narrow grip pull-down.** Using a wide grip brings in the latissimus dorsi muscles more as synergists; using a narrow grip brings the pectorals into the action more.

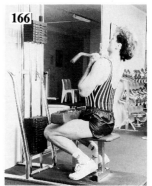

II. Triceps

1. Barbell triceps extension (fig. 167)

Uses: Works the length of the triceps.

Description: This movement can be carried out in the standing or lying position. The elbows should be kept stationary with the upper arm perpendicular to the floor. Lower the weight slowly by bending the elbows and lowering the weight past the head. Raise by straightening the elbows, but keep the arms at an angle in the finished position to keep tension on the triceps.

Special considerations
• beginners should place the feet on the bench to avoid excessive back arching;
• take care not to over-arch the back in the standing position;
• use of an 'easy curl' bar will take the strain off the forearms.

Variations
• **Wide/narrow grip tricep extension.** A wider grip works the long head of the triceps more. A narrow grip involves the 2 shorter heads of the triceps more.
• **Standing triceps extension.** In the standing position, cheating is possible and hence more weight can be added.

Other exercises

2. Dumbell triceps extension (fig. 168)

Uses: Develops the outer triceps while allowing for differences in arm strength. The dumbell action is most suited to females who generally have less upper-body strength.

Description: The movement is carried out in the prone position as with the barbell extension, except that the palms are turned inward, stressing the outer triceps. The arms should not be returned to the perpendicular in order to keep the stress on the triceps.

Variations
• **Single arm lying dumbell extension** (fig. 169). The action with a single arm tends to isolate the triceps more.
• **Lying cross body extension** (fig. 170). Instead of extending the arm behind the head, this is bent across the body while keeping the upper arm stable.

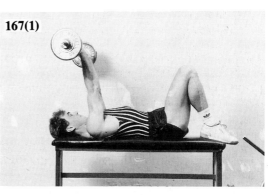

167(1)

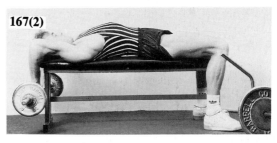

167(2)

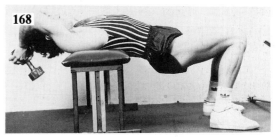

168

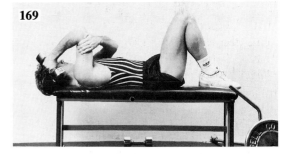

169

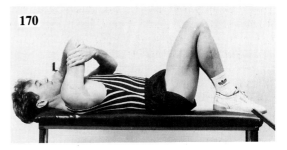

170

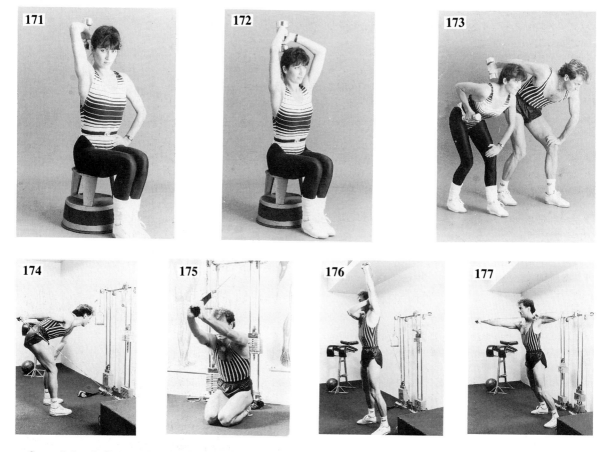

• **Seated dumbell extention.** This can be done with one arm (fig. 171) or with both arms (fig. 172). Using a single arm tends to result in a greater separation of the tricep heads.

3. Tricep kick-back (fig. 173)

Uses: Works the long head of the triceps and the upper portion of the triceps as a whole.

Description: While bending over to increase the gravitational effect, bend the weighted arm and raise the elbow to shoulder level, then straighten the arm while twisting the wrist so the thumb points upwards. The elbow can be kept in the same position or moved to bring in the long head of the triceps more.

Special considerations

• In order to keep the movement strict, the upper arm should remain stable; however, some movement of the upper arm can bring the long head of the triceps more into action as this runs across the shoulder joint;

• Do not use momentum to raise the arm.

Variations

• **Cable kick-back** (fig. 174). Using a cable provides a greater tension through the full range of movement.

4. Cable extension (fig. 175)

Uses: Works the triceps under continuous tension.

Description: The exercise can be carried out in a kneeling or standing position depending on comfort. Face away from the cable and extend the arms while keeping the upper arms stable.

Variations

• **One arm cable extension** (fig. 176). Using each arm singly allows the effort to be concentrated on that arm. The working arm should be held stable by the non-working arm.

• **Cable punches** (fig. 177). Facing away from the cables and in an upright position punch forwards. This is a useful exercise for those involved in sports using explosive upper-body actions.

5. Tricep push-down (fig. 178)

Uses: Works the triceps through the full range of movement.

Description: Cables or a lat pull-down machine are needed for this exercise. The elbows should be kept steady. Avoiding a forward bending of the body, straighten the arms at the elbows until these are almost locked, then release slowly to the bent-arm position.

Variations

• **Inclined push-down.** An incline bench can be angled towards cables or a pull-down machine to work the triceps through an unusual angle.

• **Reverse grip push-downs.** With the palms turned upwards, the push-down becomes a pull-down, which tends to stress the inner triceps more.

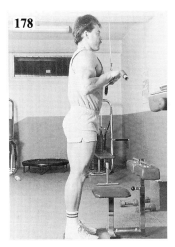

178

6. Dips (fig. 179)

Uses: A good compound exercise which develops thickness in the triceps.

Description: This is one of the best all-round upper body exercises using the chest, arms and upper back. However, it is often not an appropriate exercise for females because of the difficulty in lifting body weight. Try to lean back while returning to the upright position to stress the triceps. Extra weight can be added to the waist in very strong individuals.

Variations

• **Hands forwards/behind the body.** With the hands forward of the body the triceps and upper back are emphasised more. With the hands behind the body, the chest and shoulders are worked more.

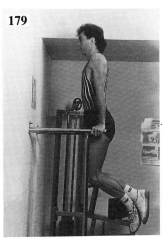

179

III. Forearms

Standard Exercise

1. Barbell wrist curl (fig. 180)

Uses: Strengthens the inside (flexor) muscles of the forearm for hand movement activities.

Description: This is an isolation movement for the forearms which are worked extensively during arm curls. Elbows should be rested on a bench or the knees as in fig. 147. The wrists are bent towards the body without elbow movement, then lowered towards the floor.

Variations

• **Behind the back wrist curls** (fig. 181). Standing

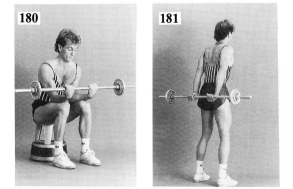

180　　181

with the bar behind the back allows a heavier weight to be used for greater strength development.

• **Dumbell wrist curls.** Using dumbells to curl the wrists results in greater isolation of the forearm muscles and allows a more natural movement of the arm.

Other exercises

2. Barbell reverse wrist curl (fig. 182)
Uses: Strengthens the outside (extensor) muscles of the forearm. Useful for the prevention of RSI, tennis elbow etc.
Description: Using an overhand grip, roll the wrists upwards with the elbows fixed. Lower the wrists to the floor.

Variations
• **Reverse wrist curls using a preacher bench.** This results in a stricter execution of the exercise.
• **Dumbell reverse wrist curls.** Using dumbells allows for a greater isolation of individual arms and therefore assists where there may be unilateral strength differences.

3. Reverse barbell curls (fig. 183)
Uses: Works the forearm extensors as well as the outer head of the biceps.

Description: With the hands shoulder-width apart, the barbell is grasped with an overhand grip and curled upwards with a curling motion of the wrist, then forearm. Lower slowly.

Variations
• **Wide/narrow grip reverse curls.** Using a wide grip emphasises the inner forearm more. Using a narrow grip emphasises the outer forearm extensors and biceps.
• **Preacher bench reverse curl.** This results in a greater strictness of movement.
• **Dumbell reverse curl.** Using dumbells allows for unilateral strength differences in the forearms.

4. Wrist rolls (fig. 184)
Uses: Strengthens the rotational movement of the forearm muscles. Good for racket sports and prevention of tennis elbow, RSI etc.
Description: With a single dumbell, roll the wrist with the forearm at right angles to the upper arm. Roll in both directions.

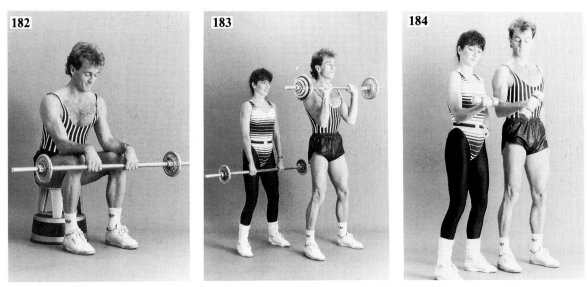

182   183   184

2.2 Exercises for the Shoulders and Upper Back

I Latissimus Dorsi, Trapezius

Standard exercise

1. Lat Pull-Down (fig. 185)
Uses: Develops and widens the upper lats. This is an alternative exercise to chin-ups for those with less upper-body strength.
Description: With a wide grip, pull the bar down to shoulder level, either behind or in front of the neck, then slowly release and straighten the arms. Do not rise off the seat during the action.

Special considerations
• If the body rises off the seat during the pull-down motion, the resistance is too great and should be reduced.

Variations
• **Narrow grip pull-down.** As the grip moves inward the action centres more on the inner portion of the upper back.
• **Reverse grip pull-down.** If the grip is reversed, the medial portion of the biceps become more involved.

Other exercises

2. Chin-up behind the neck (fig. 186)
Uses: Develops the upper back, trapezius and arms. Excellent for rowing, swimming and strength sports.
Description: The standard chin-up involves pulling the body to the bar so the back of the neck touches the bar. The feet should be crossed so the legs are not used for momentum. Lower the body slowly.

Variations
• **Wide/narrow grip front chins** (fig. 187). A wide grip involves more of the chest, allows a greater range of motion and enables some cheating to help through fatigue. Narrow grip chins can be carried out on a straight bar or with double handles (fig. 188) for a more natural hand action. The action emphasises serratus as well as lats.

3. Bent over barbell row (fig. 189)
Uses: Works the upper back and arms and helps thicken the lats. This is a useful exercise for swimming and rowing sports.
Description: With feet apart and knees slightly bent, raise the weight to touch the upper abs without cheating with the lower back. Lower slowly.

Special considerations
• This exercise should not be carried out by beginners or those with back problems;
• do not lock the knees, but keep partly flexed.

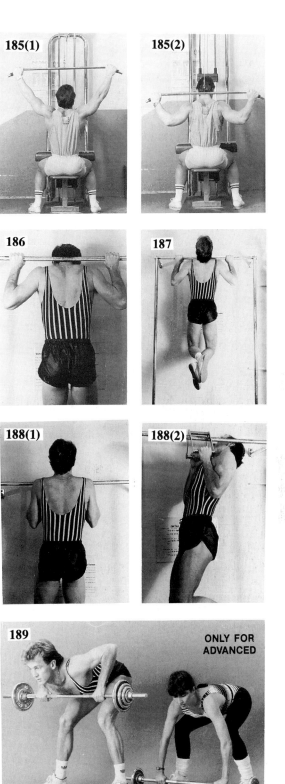

ONLY FOR ADVANCED

Variations

• **T bar row** (fig. 190). The same action can be carried out with a T bar.

• **Bent over row on bench** (fig. 191). Standing on a bench to carry out the movement allows a greater pre-stretch of the arms and lats, particularly with large weight plates which can move below toe level.

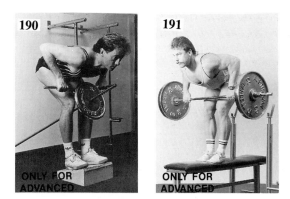

4. Bent over dumbell row (fig. 192)

Uses: Works the lats independently and allows for greater unilateral differences in strength. Using barbells makes the exercise easier for the inexperienced and less strong.

Description: The movement can be carried out standing, as in fig. 192, or seated as in fig. 193. Bring the hands up to the chest either together or alternately. Lower the weight slowly.

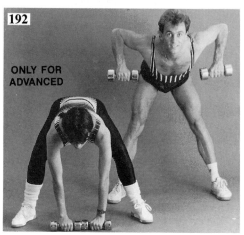

Special considerations

• Hold the upper back steady and keep the lower back flat by locking the pelvis.

• Make sure the knees are slightly flexed.

Variations

• **One arm dumbell row** (fig. 194). Rest the non-active arm on a bench, chair back etc., so the back is supported. Using arms independently isolates each side of the upper back and allows the weight to be lifted higher, thereby causing more muscle action.

• **Kneeling one arm cross-over dumbell row** (fig. 195). From a kneeling position pass the dumbell across the body and raise to shoulder height. This can be a useful upper-back exercise for aerobic classes.

• **Lying dumbell row** (fig. 196). Lying face down on a bench makes the movement more strict so that cheating is difficult. This is a useful way for beginners to learn the exercise.

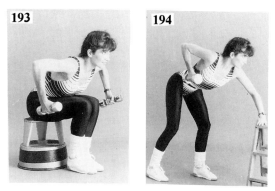

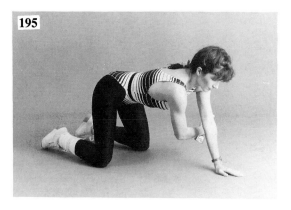

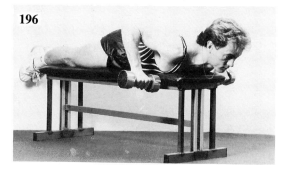

- **Lying reverse flyes** (fig. 197). From the face-down position, the arms are abducted as far as possible. This works the posterior deltoids, rhomboids and lats.

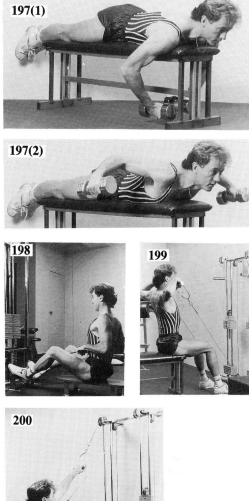

5. Seated cable row (fig. 198)
Uses: Strengthens the upper back and helps develop thickness in the lats.
Description: While seated with the knees slightly bent, pull the weight towards the abdomen without bending backwards significantly. The aim is to try to bring the shoulder blades together.

Variations
- **Reverse grip seated row.** By turning the palms of the hands upwards and pulling towards the body, the biceps are brought more into the action.
- **Single or double handed seated cable row from below** (fig. 199). While seated in front of the cables, raise the arms to shoulder level. This allows the arms to be separated and hence causes a greater contraction of the latissimus dorsi muscles. In the upright seated position as in fig. 166, deltoids are also involved in the action.
- **Single or double handed seated cable row from above** (fig. 200). The arms are pulled down towards the body either independently or together. This action works the lower lats and biceps and as with the row from below (fig. 199), is an ideal exercise for canoeing or rowing.

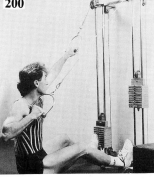

6. Bent over cable cross-overs (fig. 201)
Uses: Works the outer lats concentrically and pectorals eccentrically. Also works the posterior deltoids.
Description: With the back bent and the knees slightly flexed, cross over the cables in front of the body and abduct the arms against the resistance. The lower back should remain stationary.

Special considerations
- This exercise should not be carried out by beginners or those with back problems;
- Make sure the knees do not lock.

Variations
- **Single arm cable rows.** Using one side of the body at a time allows a greater stretch and concentrates the action more on the side of movement.

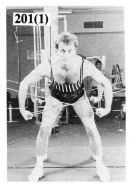
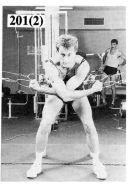

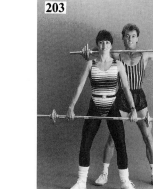
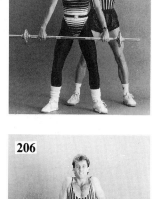
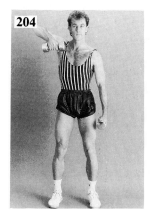
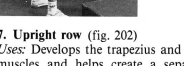
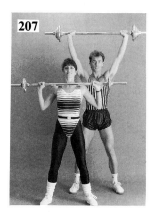

7. Upright row (fig. 202)

Uses: Develops the trapezius and anterior deltoid muscles and helps create a separation between deltoids and pectorals.

Description: Grasp the barbell in an overhand grip and with the knees slightly bent, raise to the chin without the aid of the lower back. Lower slowly.

Variations

• **Wide-grip upright row** (fig. 203). With a wide grip the medial deltoids are emphasised more.

• **Single-arm dumbell row** (fig. 204). The use of dumbells allows for unilateral strength differences between arms.

• **Single arm cable upright row** (fig. 205). Cables allow a greater range of movement in the trapezius, and cater for arm strength differences.

8. Shrugs (fig. 206)

Uses: Develops trapezius and is therefore useful for protection of the neck such as in contact sports.

Description: Using an overhand grip on the bar and with the weight held at arms length, raise the shoulders to touch the ears. The shoulders can be rolled back on the downward movement to bring the upper back into the movement. With a heavy weight, one hand may grasp the bar in an underhand grip.

Variations

• **Dumbell shrugs.** Using dumbells enables a heavier weight to be lifted and allows a greater range of motion as the palms can be turned inward.

II Deltoids

Standard exercise

1. Military press (fig. 207)

Uses: Works deltoids and triceps.

Description: The hands should be slightly wider than shoulder-width apart. With the bar held in front of the neck, raise the weight to full arm extension without arching the lower back. Lower slowly.

• This is not a good exercise for beginners because of the danger to the lower back;
• Keep the back straight. If an arch occurs, this indicates the weight is too heavy.

Variations

• **Press behind the neck** (fig. 208). Starting with the weight behind, instead of in front of the neck, brings the medial deltoids and trapezius more into the action.

• **Seated press** (fig. 209). If a back support is used, the movement is made more strict and safer for the back.

• **Machine press** (fig. 210). Press machines are made by several manufacturers. These are better for the inexperienced to learn the correct lifting techniques.

• **Single arm dumbell press** (fig. 211). Using dumbells helps compensate for unilateral strength differences.

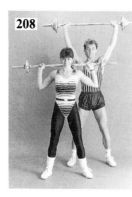
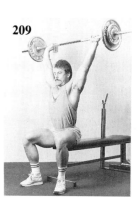
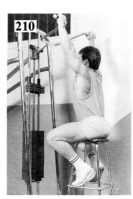
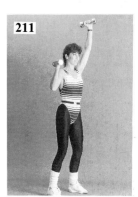

Other exercises

2. Clean (fig. 212)

Uses: An excellent and under-rated compound exercise which works the back, shoulders, legs and arms.

Description: The feet should be shoulder-width apart and the knees slightly bent. Lift the weight off the floor with an overhand grip and hands spaced slightly wider than the feet. Roll the forearms and curl the bar to shoulder level in one action while standing straight up. Hold in this position with the elbows tucked in and under to support the weight. Lower to arms length, then the floor in 2 actions.

Special considerations:
• Avoid back arching;
• Lower the weight slowly; do not drop suddenly from the chest to arms length position.

Variations

• **Dumbell clean** (*see* fig. 212). Dumbell use allows for more independent arm action and a greater involvement of the biceps.

• **Clean with press.** The weight can be pressed from the chest position to above the head before it is lowered. This should only be carried out by experienced weight lifters.

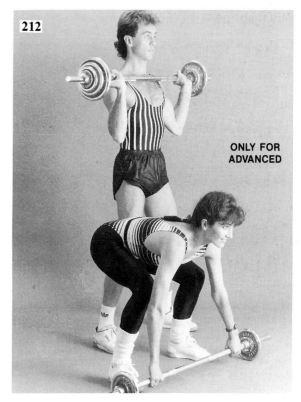

ONLY FOR ADVANCED

3. Dumbell lateral raise (fig. 213)

Uses: Develops and strengthens deltoids and is therefore ideal for sports requiring shoulder strength.

Description: With a dumbell in each hand, elbows slightly bent and palms facing inwards, raise the arms laterally to shoulder level. Keep the elbows bent to take the pressure off the joint. Movement past shoulder level brings in the trapezius muscle and means that a heavier weight could be used and just raised to shoulder level. Lower slowly and start each movement from a completely stationary position.

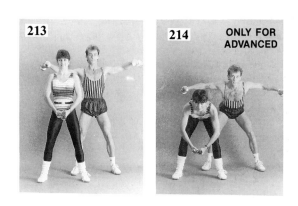

Special considerations
- Avoid arching of the back;
- Keep the knees slightly flexed;
- Keep the elbows slightly bent to avoid excessive pressure on the joint.

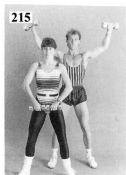
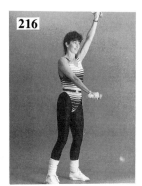

Variations
- **Seated lateral raise.** The movement is made more strict from the seated position.
- **Bent over lateral raise** (fig. 214). With the body flexed at the waist, the posterior head of the deltoids is brought more into action.
- **Forward dumbell raise** (fig. 215). Raising the arms to the front of the body emphasises the anterior deltoids.
- **Single-arm forward dumbell raise** (fig. 216). Allows for strength differences between arms.

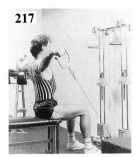
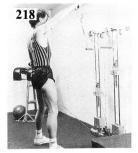

4. Cable lateral raise (fig. 217)

Uses: Allows for unilateral development of the deltoids under continuous tension.

Description: The action is similar to that using dumbells. It can be carried out in the seated or standing position. The back should be kept straight and the cable raised to just above shoulder level. Lower the weight slowly.

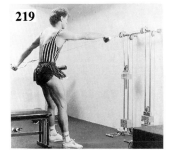

Variations
- **Forward cable raise** (fig. 218) works the anterior deltoids more.
- **Rear cable raise** (fig. 219) works the posterior deltoids in an action simulating a cross-country skiing movement.

5. One-arm cross cable laterals (fig. 220)

Uses: Works and isolates the medial and posterior heads of the deltoids.

Description: With the arm down and across the front of the body, pull the cable to the point where the hand is level with the shoulder. Twist the wrist downwards as the arm is raised. Lower slowly.

Special considerations
• Do not use the momentum of the body to raise the weight;
• the movement should be carried out slowly and not in a jerky fashion.

Variations
• **One arm cross cable laterals from the rear** (fig. 221). The starting position is similar to the front of the body action except that the cable is now held behind the back. Abducting the arm in this fashion puts more emphasis on the anterior and medial deltoids.

6. Upright dumbell flyes (fig. 222)

Uses: Develops strength and stamina in the deltoids for strength-endurance activities such as windsurfing, sailing, etc.

Description: In the upright seated position with the dumbells in front of the chest and arms level with the chest, abduct the arms as far as possible. Return to the start position without lowering the weight.

Special considerations
• Avoid arching the back; back support is recommended where possible;
• Do not 'throw' the arms behind the shoulders in the abducted position.

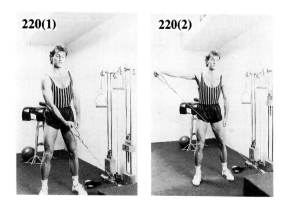

220(1)   220(2)

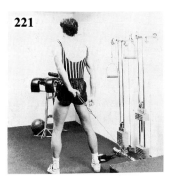

221

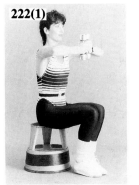

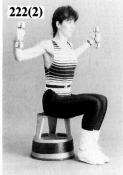

222(1)   222(2)

2.3 Exercises for the Chest and Middle Back

I Pectorals

Standard exercise

1. Bench Press (fig. 223)
Uses: Increases the size of the chest and the strength of the arms, chest and shoulders.
Description: This is one of the best upper-body compound exercises available. Beginners should place the feet on the bench for support. Experienced lifters on the other hand may need to keep the feet on the floor for extra support with a heavy weight. The arms should be wide enough apart so the forearms are perpendicular to the floor in the bottom position. Extend the arms while raising the weight above the body and then lower slowly.

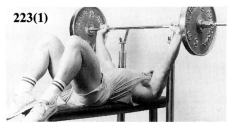

223(1)

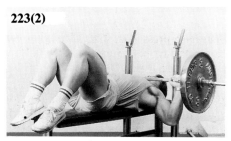

223(2)

Special considerations
• Ensure that the weight is not 'thrown' in the upward action by excessive arching of the back and use of the feet in the action;
• Return the weight as low to the chest as possible, but do not let it rest on the chest before recommencing the upwards movement.

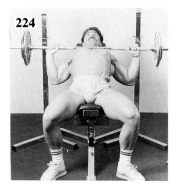

224

Variations
• **Incline bench press** (fig. 224). Working on an incline places the emphasis more on the superior pectorals and deltoids.
• **Decline bench press** (fig. 225). Working on a decline places the emphasis more on the inferior pectorals.
• **Machine bench press** (fig. 226). This is an excellent way for beginners to learn the strict action of the movement.
• **Wide/narrow grip bench press.** A wide grip on the bar puts the emphasis more on the lateral pectorals and pectoralis minor. A narrow grip puts the emphasis more on the medial pectorals, and helps develop the 'cleavage' or split between the pectorals.
• **Thumbs under grip bench press.** With the thumb wrapped around the bar in line with the fingers, the emphasis is put more on the triceps.

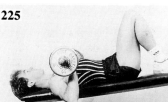

225

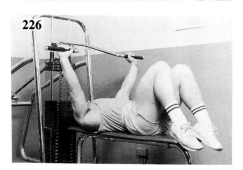

226

Other exercises

2. Dumbell Bench Press (fig. 227)

Uses: Develops pectorals, deltoids and triceps and allows for unilateral weaknesses and injuries in the arms and shoulders.

Description: The arms can be worked independently or together to raise the weight as in the barbell press. Dumbells allow a greater stretch of the pectorals and shoulders in the action.

Variations

• **Decline dumbell press** (fig. 228). Carrying out the action on a decline bench puts more emphasis independently on the inferior portion of the pectoral muscles.

• **Incline dumbell press.** Carrying out the action on an incline puts more emphasis independently on the superior portion of the pectoral muscles.

3. Dumbell pullovers (fig. 229)

Uses: Helps to expand the chest capacity and

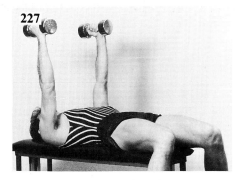

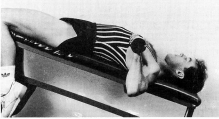

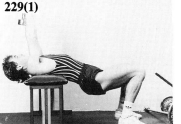

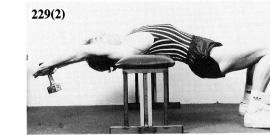

develop the rib cage. Good for aiding breathing difficulty problems.

Description: Lie across a bench with a single dumbell grasped in both hands and both palms pressing against the top plate. Lower the weight slowly over the head until the arms are straight and drop the hips to the floor at the same time.

Special considerations

• Do not overarch the back;

• Do not drop the weight from the overhead position; return the weight to the lap and sit up before placing back on the floor.

Variations

• **Bent arm pullover** (fig. 230). Bending the arms allows a greater weight to be lifted with less strain. More emphasis is also put on the serratus muscles in this action.

• **Barbell pullover** (fig. 231). This requires more co-ordination between the arms.

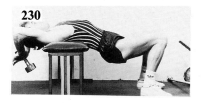

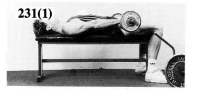

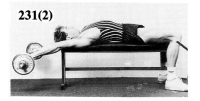

4. Dumbell flyes (fig. 232)

Uses: One of the best isolation exercises for pectoral development.

Description: On a flat bench with the arms extended above the body and the palms facing inwards, lower the weights slowly out to each side as far as possible without arching the back. Keep the elbows slightly bent and return to the starting position with a quicker movement.

Special considerations
• Beginners should keep the knees bent and feet on the bench for back support; with more experience and more weight, the feet may be kept on the floor for more support.

Variations
• **Incline flyes** (fig. 233). Carrying the movement out on an incline puts the emphasis more on the superior portion of the pectorals.
• **Decline flyes** (fig. 234). Carrying the movement out on a decline puts the emphasis more on the inferior portion of the pectorals.

5. Pec dec flyes (fig. 235)

Uses: Develops definition in the pectoral muscles. This is one of the most popular gym machines available.

Description: The machine should be taken to the full extension in order to get maximum contraction potential. Keep the back straight and the upper arms parallel to the floor. Draw the arms together and squeeze in the front of the chest. Return slowly.

6. Cable cross-overs (fig. 236)

Uses: Develops definition in the medial pectorals.

Description: Using cables, grasp a handle in each hand. While bent slightly forwards, draw the hands together and allow them to cross. Slowly release until the arms are level with the shoulders.

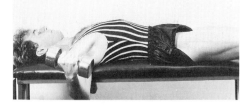

232

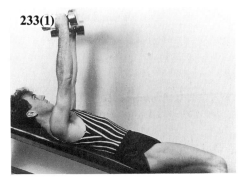

233(1)

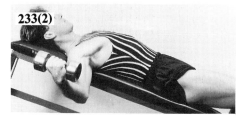

233(2)

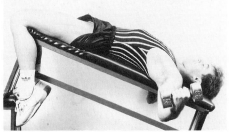

234

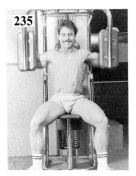

235

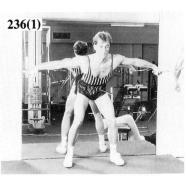

236(1)

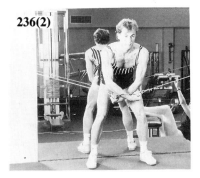

236(2)

7. Pull-down in front of neck (fig. 237)
Uses: Works the lower lats and pectorals as well as biceps and forearms.
Description: Using a lat pull-down machine with a wide handgrip, pull the weight to touch the front of the chest. Release slowly.

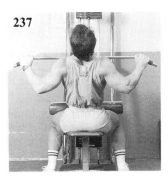

2.4 Exercises for the Legs

I Quadriceps

Standard exercise

1. The squat (fig. 238)
Uses: Builds strength and mass in the thighs.
Description: With the weight centred firmly on the shoulders, the action is to descend to a level where the thighs are parallel to the floor. Exceeding this point puts excessive strain on the ligaments of the knee and back of the patella which is not justified for the extra benefit gained. Descend slowly and accelerate in the upwards action.

Special considerations
• The weight should be centred at all times over the middle of the feet;
• Keep the head up and back straight during the movement.
• Do not bounce out of the bottom position;
• Keep the feet flat on the floor to increase achilles flexibility;
• Ensure that the knees do not turn inwards with the action;
• Do not lean forwards in the movement.

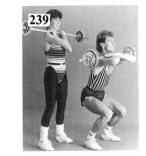

Variations
• **Front squats** (fig. 239). Holding the weight in front of the body puts the emphasis more on the anterior and inferior portions of the thighs.
• **Narrow stance squat** (fig. 240). With the feet close together, more emphasis is put on the outer quadriceps.
• **Wide stance squat** (fig. 241). With the feet wider apart and the toes turned out, the inner thighs are worked more.
• **Machine squats** (fig. 242). A squat machine is useful for beginners to learn the correct action of the movement.

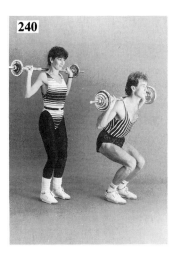

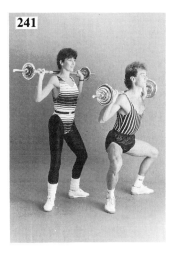

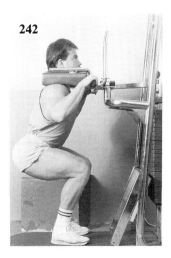

Other exercises

2. The lunge (fig. 243)
Uses: Develops and strengthens the anterior quadriceps.
Description: This form of leg action is probably best for those such as females and beginners who may use light weights. With the weight on the shoulders, step forwards until the trailing knee almost touches the floor. Return to the starting position and repeat with the opposite leg.

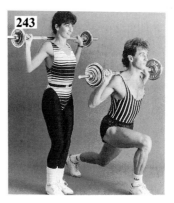

3. Leg extension (fig. 244)
Uses: Isolates the biceps femoris and vastus medialis at the front of the thigh for extra strength and definition. A good pre-exhaustion exercise to be combined with the squat.
Description: Using a leg extension machine, extend the legs fully, then lower slowly.

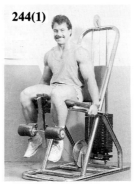 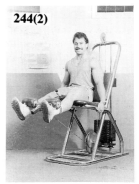

Special considerations
• Avoid 'throwing' the weight up with the legs;
• Support the back with the hands and do not overarch with the back.

Variations
• **Toes out/toes in leg extension.** Pointing the toes out works the vastus medialis more and is useful in rehabilitation of medial ligament damage. Pointing the toes in works the vastus lateralis more and is useful for rehabilitation of lateral ligament damage.

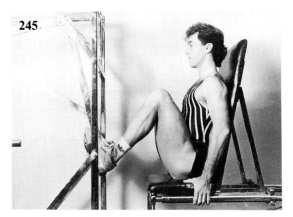

4. Leg press (fig. 245)
Uses: Helps build strength in the thighs, placing less stress on the back than with some other leg exercises.
Description: In the leg press machine (different angles are possible), press out with the thighs against the weight until the legs are straight. Support the back and keep the hands by the sides during the action.

5. Hack squat (fig. 246)
Uses: Develops the inferior portion of the quadriceps with the pressure taken off the back.
Description: Using a hack squat machine, tuck the shoulders under the padded bars and take hold of the handles while in the crouched position. Stand quickly using the thighs to take the weight until the legs are straight. Return slowly to the starting position.

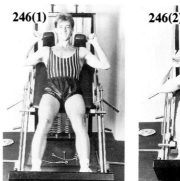

6. Step ups (fig. 247)

Uses: To develop the strength of the thighs in a stair climbing action.

Description: With a weight on the shoulders, step up onto a bench or step no higher than a position where the thigh is parallel to the floor. Step up with the other foot until standing on the step, then step down one foot at a time. Change the foot for stepping up and repeat the action.

7. Cable leg press (fig. 248)

Uses: Works quadriceps and hip flexors unilaterally with continuous tension. A good beginner's hip and thigh exercise.

Description: With overhead cable behind the body, attach a cable strap to the foot of one leg and press out until the leg is straight. Slowly release. Keep the weight on the elbows to avoid back problems.

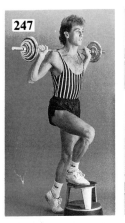
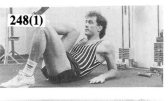
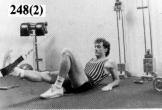
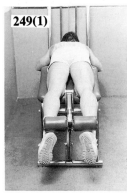

II Hamstrings

Standard exercise

1. Leg curl (fig. 249)

Uses: Develops strength in the hamstrings.

Description: Lying on a leg-curl machine, hook the feet under the level mechanism and with hips fixed on the bench, curl the legs as far as possible. Do not arch the back or fling the weight with momentum. Lower slowly from the upright position.

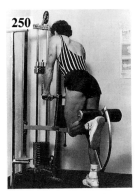
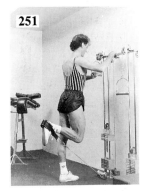

Variations

• **Standing leg curl** (fig. 250). Standing enables unilateral isolation of the hamstring muscles with greater emphasis through the range of movement because of the lack of gravitational assistance.

• **Cable leg curl** (fig. 251). This provides continuous resistance through the full range of motion.

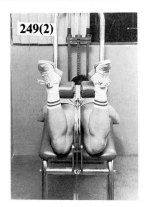

Other exercises

2. Leg cable pull-down (fig. 252)
Uses: Works the hip extensors and the superior portion of the hamstrings, which often cause problems in sprinting and other explosive sports.
Description: Lying away from an above-pulley cable system, hook one foot into a foot strap with the leg straight and flexed at the hip. Push down until the leg is straight, then slowly return.

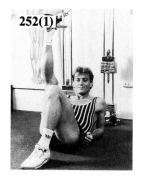
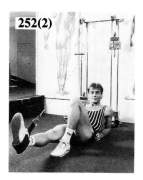

III Hip Flexors and Extensors, Leg Abductors and Adductors

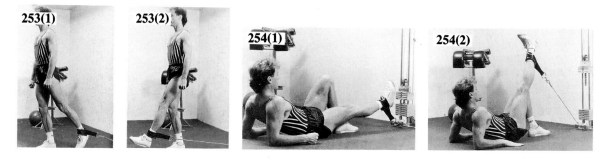

1. Cable hip flexion (fig. 253)
Uses: Strengthens forward hip flexors.
Description: Standing facing away from a low pulley system with one foot in a foot strap and leg straight, flex the hip so the leg is forced away from the body, then slowly release. Repeat with the other leg.

Variations

• **Lying cable hip flexion** (fig. 254). The lying position allows more support for the back.

• **Supine cable hip flexion** (fig. 255). This strengthens the hip flexors from a greater pre-stretched position.

• **Bent-leg cable hip flexion** (fig. 256). Bending the leg means the superior quadriceps muscles as well as the hip flexors will be emphasised more.

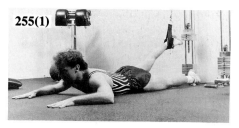

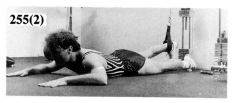

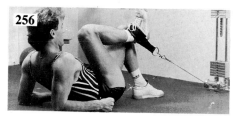

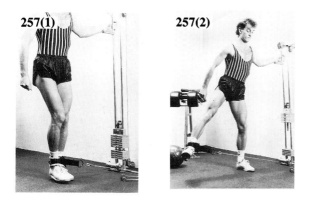

257(1)   257(2)

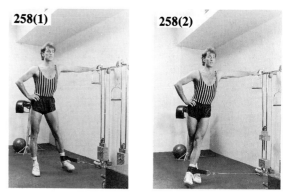

258(1)   258(2)

2. Cable leg abduction (fig. 257)
Uses: Strengthens the outside of the thigh.
Description: Standing side-on to a low pulley system, abduct the outside leg with weight attached as far as possible. Slowly release and repeat with the opposite leg.

3. Cable leg adduction (fig. 258)
Uses: Strengthens the inside of the thigh.
Description: Standing side-on to a low pulley system with the cable attached to the inside leg, adduct the leg across the body as far as possible. Slowly release and repeat with the opposite leg.

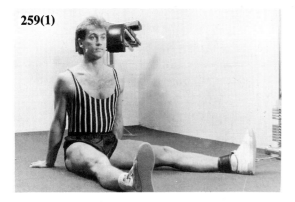

259(1)

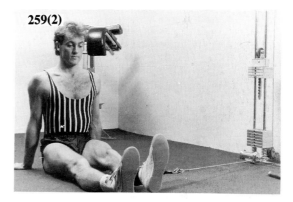

259(2)

Variations
• **Seated cable leg adduction** (fig. 259). This adds variety to the movement.

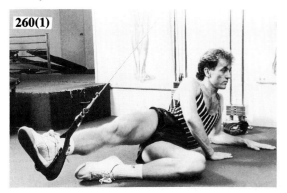

260(1)

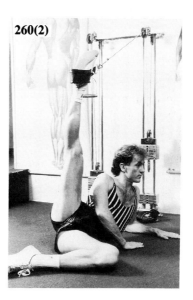

260(2)

• **Lying side cable leg adduction** (fig. 260). Lying on the side strengthens the adductors from a greater pre-stretched position.

73

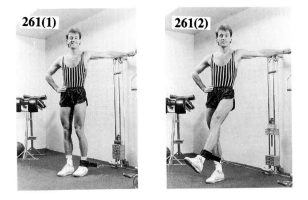

261(1)   261(2)

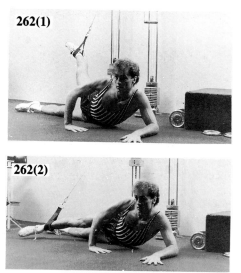

262(1)

262(2)

• **Forward facing cable leg adduction** (fig. 261). At an angle, hip flexors as well as adductors are brought into the movement more.

• **Forward lying cable leg adduction** (fig. 262). This achieves the action of fig. 261 from a greater pre-stretched position.

IV Gastrocnemius (Calves)

Standard exercise

1. Standing heel raise (fig. 263)
Uses: Develops and strengthens the calves.
Description: With a weight on the shoulders and feet flat on the floor or heels extended over a block, raise the body on the toes as far as possible. Return to the starting position.

Variations
• **Heel raise machine** (fig. 264). The calf machine allows greater weight to be used and ensures strictness of movement in the action.

• **One-legged heel raise** (fig. 265). This works the calves unilaterally with greater pressure on the individual calf.

• **Seated heel raise** (fig. 266). In a seated position and with the weight resting on the knees, the lower and outer area of the calves are emphasised.

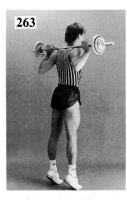

263

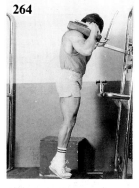

264

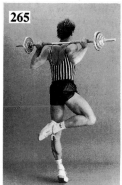

265

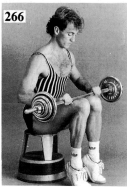

266

74

2.5 Exercises for the Abdomen and Lower Back

I Rectus Abdominus, External and Internal Obliques

Note: Research has shown that the best forms of abdominal exercise are carried out on a flat surface without the use of extra weights. Holding or locking the feet, such as on an abdominal sit-up board, brings in muscle groups other than the abdominals (e.g. hip flexors such as iliopsoas) and hence reduces the effectiveness of the exercise for the abdominals.

For this reason most abdominal exercises are covered in Section 1 (Aerobic Floor Classes section) of this book. Some extra abdominal exercises using weights or equipment are shown below.

Standard exercise

1. Crunch (fig. 267)
Uses: Strengthens and tones rectus abdominus.
Description: With hips flexed and heels pushed to the floor, raise the shoulders as far off the ground as possible. Hands should be held lightly to the side of the head or ears to avoid neck injury by pulling the head forwards.

Special considerations
• Do not raise the feet off the ground;
• Do not hold the feet down;
• Do not jerk the back in the upward motion.

Variations (Using weights)
• **Jack-knife crunch** (fig. 268). Crunching up, touch the toes of extended legs. This involves inferior rectus abdominus more in the exercise.

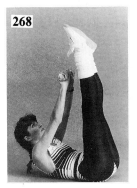

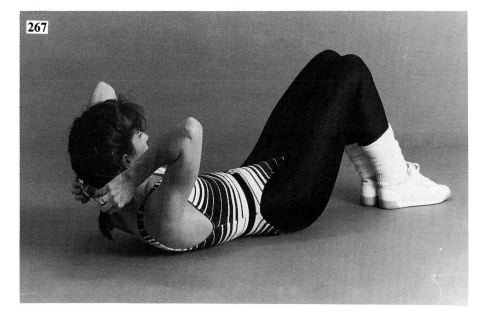

Other exercises

2. Side sit-up and twist (fig. 269)

Uses: Works rectus abdominus and obliques.

Description: Here the exerciser's legs are held at the knees and the motion is to twist during the movement from the side lying position to face the partner. This is an advanced exercise and requires strong abdominals.

3. Hip flexion (fig. 270)

Uses: Works superior rectus abdominus and hip flexors.

Description: While in a hanging position on a hip flexion machine, raise the knees as high as possible to the chest. The knees should be bent to take the

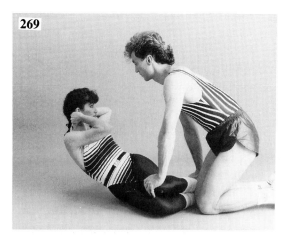

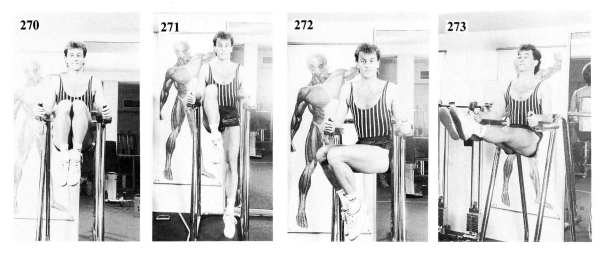

pressure off the deeper hip flexor muscles. Lower the legs slowly.

Variations

• **One-legged hip flexion** (fig. 271). Using legs alternately helps isolate the lateral portion of the abdominals.

• **Hip flexion with twist** (fig. 272). Twisting works the obliques as well as the rectus abdominus muscles.

• **Straight-legged hip flexion** (fig. 273). This works the deeper hip flexor muscles for sports in which greater strength of these may be required e.g. skiing.

4. Cable crunch (fig. 274)

Uses: Strengthens abdominals and causes separation of serratus muscles of the chest.

Description: Holding a high cable system from above and without moving the arms, crunch the

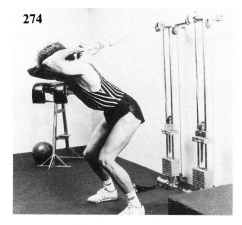

upper body towards the lower body. Try not to bring the legs or arms into the motion, working only the abdominals.

II Erector Spinae Group

Standard exercise

1. Good morning (fig. 275)
Uses: Strengthens the muscles of the lower back.
Description: With a weight on the shoulders, knees slightly bent and feet shoulder-width apart, bend forwards until the upper body is parallel to the ground. Keep the head up and back straight. Slowly rise to the upright position.

This is an advanced exercise and should only be carried out where there is no indication of back injury.

2. Bent leg dead lift (fig. 276)
Uses: Good compound exercise stressing the lower back.
Description: With knees slightly bent and feet shoulder-width apart, bend to pick up a weight. The grip can be overhand or one hand over and one hand under the bar for better balance. Rise to the standing position using only the back and legs. Return the weight slowly to the floor.

Variations
• **Straight leg dead lift.** This stretches the hamstrings in the movement, but should only be carried out by advanced lifters.

3. Back extension (fig. 277)
Uses: Works lower back muscles.
Description: This exercise is often described as 'hyperextension' which it should not be. In an extension machine with the body facing down, raise the upper body until it is level or *slightly* higher than the lower limbs. Hold and return slowly to the starting position.

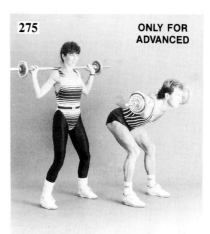

275 **ONLY FOR ADVANCED**

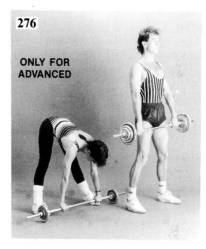

276

ONLY FOR ADVANCED

Variations
• **Back extension with twist.** Twisting alternately to each side on the upward action brings in the quadratus muscles of the lower back.

277(1)

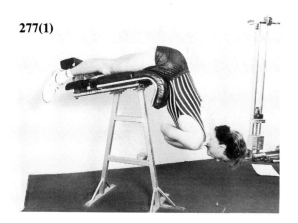

277(2)

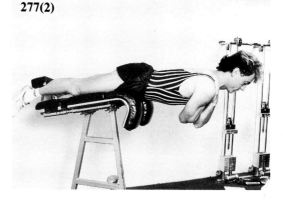

Part C: Flexibility Training Exercises

Background

Muscles are the body's means of movement. Skeletal muscles, or those attached to bones, generally run across at least one joint. Some, such as the biceps, run across 2 joints.

When a muscle contracts and shortens, which is its major function, this causes one bone to be pulled towards another, decreasing the angle between the bones at the joint. In the case of the biceps, the forearm is pulled towards the shoulder, decreasing the angle at the elbow.

A muscle therefore needs strength. But it also needs length. If a muscle is long but not strong, little force will be able to be exerted in a movement. If, on the other hand it is strong, but not long, muscle damage can occur, particularly in a fast movement involving an opposing or 'antagonist' muscle.

Because muscles work in pairs, it is also not possible to have strength without length. A short muscle will mean that the agonist is not able to contract fully without resistance from the shortened antagonist. If a muscle is continually contracted, friction may be caused in the opposing muscle, resulting in either muscle tears, or chronic injury, such as tendinitis. The connection of the muscle onto the bone (epiphysis), can also be irritated in the case of a shortened muscle, causing 'epiphysitis', or in the case of the front of the lower leg, 'shin splints'.

A further reason for stretching is that natural muscle shrinkage with age tends to result in problems of stiffness and lack of mobility. Hence it seems that many of the problems associated with this in old age can be improved by a regular program of stretching. This is particularly so with problems of the lower back caused by inflexible lower back and hamstring muscles.

The main reasons for stretching are:

(a) to decrease the risk of injury;

(b) to enable full development of opposing muscle groups;

(c) to increase mobility and decrease problems of lack of mobility with increasing age.

Other associated reasons are:

- to improve relaxation and decrease stress;
- to enable improvements in posture;
- to decrease pain and mobility problems associated with ailments such as arthritis and chronic muscle tension;
- to improve blood circulation by allowing a free flow of blood through relaxed muscles of the body.

1.1 What Stretching is Not

While stretching is an integral part of overall fitness, it is not itself a means of developing aerobic fitness or burning body fat. This can only come from a program utilising aerobic energy.

Any stretching program then, should be combined with an aerobic program, rather than take its place. Certain oriental exercise forms such as yoga and tai chi are extremely good forms of flexibility training. But they have little effect on aerobic capacity. If weight loss occurs, this can generally be attributed to the relaxation effects of the exercise which might result in less food being eaten.

1.2 When to Stretch

While few exercise specialists would argue about the importance of stretching, there has been a great deal of controversy about when and how to stretch properly.

In the early days of aerobics classes, it was thought important to stretch all the major muscle groups before involving them in any form of strenuous aerobic activity. But this had some disadvantages because the sudden extension of a 'cold' muscle could cause strains or tears.

The fashion then became to stretch following a general total body warm-up such as a brisk walk or light jog. In the early 1980s however, the value of this approach was questioned by San Diego sports medicine specialist, Dr Richard Dominguez, who suggested that stretching as part of the total body warm-up i.e. in the ranges of motion to be used, was a more economical and safer way of preparing muscles for action.

This type of 'Range of Motion' (ROM) stretching has now become an accepted way of commencing an aerobics class. Static stretching on the other hand is regarded as an appropriate way of maintaining muscle integrity after an exercise workout.

In a situation where only flexibility exercises are being carried out e.g. such as in a 'stretch' or 'mobility' class, it is important to ensure that muscles are warm before they are stretched.

1.3 How to Stretch

There are 4 main types of stretching now in vogue, 3 of which are commonly used in modern exercise programs:

1. Ballistic stretching is bounce stretching, where the muscle is taken to the end of its range of motion, and then overstretched by bouncing. This used to be a common form of stretching, but has now been discarded because of a knowledge of the intra-muscular damage that may occur as a result of the 'stretch reflex'.

The stretch reflex: Muscle fibres contain sensory nerve endings within the muscle called *muscle spindles* whose main function is to send messages back from the muscle to inform about its state of stretch.

If the muscle is stretched, distortion of the central part of the muscle spindle causes the stretch reflex to automatically come into play to contract the muscle, thus avoiding damage through tearing.

This is similar to suddenly pulling a piece of elastic taut and then letting it go.

The amount and rate of contraction elicited from the stretch reflex are proportional to the amount and rate of stretching. Hence, the faster and more forceful the stretch, the faster and more forceful the reflex contraction of the stretched muscle and thus the likelihood of the muscle tearing—particularly in an untrained muscle.

Bouncing, or 'ballistic' actions in exercise are therefore not recommended because of the potential damage caused by the stretch reflex in the average (untrained) person.

But the stretch reflex is only part of what is called the 'myotatic' response (*myo* = muscle; *tasis* = stretch). A second reflex action called the *inverse stretch reflex* originates from sensory nerves (called 'Golgi tendon organs'), which are found in the tendon of a muscle.

The Golgi tendon organs respond more to increases in the muscle tension and to forceful contraction and extreme stretch rather than muscle length, and are thus brought into play when a muscle is stretched to its full extent and held for 6 seconds or more. It seems that these nerves then initiate a reaction which causes the antagonist (or opposite) muscle to that being stretched to relax, thus allowing the muscle to be stretched without damage.

Bouncing (ballistic) actions thus cause resistance in the muscle spindle due to the stretch reflex, and are not extended for long enough to gain the benefits of the inverse stretch reflex. For this reason, bouncing style exercises (such as those initially used on the 'Jane Fonda Tapes'), are now thought to be not only wrong, but potentially dangerous *for the untrained athlete.*

Ballistic stretching exercises may be important in the well-conditioned athlete who may require ballistic actions in his/her sport. But in this case such actions should be preceded by one of the other forms of stretching outlined below.

2. Static stretching involves the gradual stretching of a muscle to a position where it is held, *without bouncing* from 10 to 30 seconds. The muscle should not be taken beyond a point of mild discomfort.

Static stretching is a safe and effective way of stretching muscles and connective tissue. Because it involves no sudden movements it does not provoke the stretch reflex as much as the ballistic method, and has a beneficial effect on the inverse stretch reflex.

Static stretching is best suited for:

- the early stages of recovery from injury;
- the cool-down phase of a vigorous exercise program.

3. PNF stretching is a form of stretching derived from physiotherapy treatment. The initials stand for *proprioceptive neuromuscular facilitation,* which simply implies that a positive training effect is facilitated in the pathways of nerves as well as the muscles.

The system was developed by 2 American physiotherapists in the 1950s to assist in the rehabilitation of muscle injury. It was adapted for general flexibility training in 1974 by Dr Laurence Holt from Dalhousie University in Canada who developed a system known as *Scientific Stretching for Sport.*

PNF stretching in its strictest form requires the lengthening of a muscle against resistance from a partner. The system can be adapted for individual use however by applying an immovable force to a stretched muscle. In this way almost any passive stretch can be converted to a form of PNF stretch, a process which Holt claims is a 10% more effective way of lengthening muscle tissue.

The stages of PNF stretching are:

(i) Statically stretch the muscle involved.
(ii) From the stretched position, isometrically contract the muscle against an immovable resistance (i.e. the ground, a bench, a partner or other muscle groups). Hold for 10 seconds.
(iii) Relax the muscle for a few seconds.
(iv) Move further into the stretched position and repeat the isometric contraction.

This technique is the method now preferred by sports physiotherapists and trainers as it actually works with the stretch reflex rather than against it, thus promoting an increase in muscle length.

The isometric exercise with the stretched muscle has a twofold effect. Firstly, the muscle to be stretched is encouraged to relax more completely after an isometric contraction, as tension in the contractile component of the muscle subsides after the muscle is contracted. In effect, this means that the muscle is more able to fully 'let go' and allow a more complete stretch.

The second effect is in the improved ability of the isometrically strengthened muscle to resist forces that may overstretch it, thus causing muscle damage.

PNF stretching is most suited for:

- recovery from injury;
- stretching in the cool-down phase of an exercise program;
- increasing the length of muscle before an athletic or sports event.

4. Range-of-motion (ROM) stretching arose out of a concern that some people tend to overstretch in the passive or PNF stretch situation. This may cause damage to muscle and tendon fibres, particularly in the case of recovery from overuse injuries, such as tendinitis.

ROM stretching which was made fashionable by American sports medicine specialist Dr Richard Dominguez, involves moving a muscle through its full range of motion, and increasing this range of motion with increasing repetitive movements. For example, to stretch the hamstring muscles at the back of the leg, one leg should be raised forwards as in a gentle kicking motion, with the kicking arc becoming greater with increasing repetitions.

ROM stretching is more suitable for:

- stretching immediately before a period of vigorous activity (such as an aerobics class);
- stretching of soft tissue structures of the neck, back and shoulders in particular.

1.4 Rules for Stretching

The following are basic principles which should be followed in any program involving stretching:

- breathe slowly, deeply and evenly;
- do not stretch to the point where breathing becomes unnatural;
- do not overstretch, particularly in the early stages;
- hold a stretch in a comfortable position; tension should subside as the stretch is held;
- warm up by walking briskly, or lightly jogging on the spot, before starting to stretch;
- concentrate on the area being stretched to ensure that a proper stretch is being felt;
- if appropriate, combine different types of stretching in the one session (e.g. static and ROM in an aerobics class).
- stretch before and after an extended exercise period;
- stretch regularly during the day (even for short periods) to improve overall flexibility.

1.5 Guidelines for Flexibility Training

The following are guidelines for flexibility training adapted from the document 'Standards and Guidelines for the Planning and Conduct of Fitness Programs' produced by the Australian Fitness Accreditation Council.

1. Stretching should be either:
(a) static;
(b) proprioceptive neuromuscular facilitation (PNF); or
(c) range of motion (ROM).

2. Bouncy, jerky (ballistic) movements should be avoided. These can be potentially hazardous, particularly with untrained muscles.

3. Stretching should progress from major joints to more specific joints. This ensures adequate support for all muscle groups involved.

4. Stretching should be carried out immediately before, after and even during an active sports event. Research has shown that up to one third of the flexibility gains from stretching can be lost in half an hour of sitting still before competition, and up to two-thirds in an hour.

5. Sport-specific flexibility should be developed by identifying the movements of the sport and training specifically in these movements.

6. Flexibility training should be regular, i.e. 3–4 times a week. Noticeable increases in flexibility with training can be achieved within 2–3 weeks. Decreases can occur almost as quickly.

7. Stretching exercises should be carried out slowly without forcing tight muscles to overstretch. If pain is felt, the muscle should be slightly relaxed until only a feeling of mild tension is felt.

8. If stretching is discontinued as a result of injury, qualified advice should be sought before flexibility training is recommenced.

9. Stretching involving hyperextension of the lower back can often aggravate minor injuries and therefore should involve special care and attention, particularly with inexperienced exercisers.

10. Pregnant women should only undertake flexibility training under supervision. During pregnancy, hormones are released which soften ligaments to make the skeletal structures of the hips and pelvis extensible for carrying an infant. This increases the hypermobility of joints, but exercises that place strain on these hypermobile joints can cause pain and chronic joint problems.

11. With PNF stretching, careful attention should be paid to the correct execution of exercises. If this is not done, the results could be counter-productive.

12. The optimal time for holding an isometric contraction in a PNF stretch is 6 seconds. Other static stretching can be held from 10–30 seconds.

13. Assess flexibility progress occasionally to ensure that one side of the body is not progressing faster than the other. This can be done through bilateral measurements or visual observations.

2. The Stretches

2.1 Stretches for the Calves and Shins

I Gastrocnemius

Standard stretch

1. The standing straight leg calf stretch *(fig. 278)*
Uses: Stretches the gastrocnemius. This is an important stretch for activities that require explosive movements such as jumping and sprinting.
Description: This is the standard exercise for stretching the upper part of the calf muscle (gastrocnemius). Lean against a wall, car etc with the back leg straight and the front leg bent. To increase the stretch, lean closer to the wall whilst ensuring the heel of the back leg remains on the ground.

Special considerations:
• Do not stand too far away from the wall
• Ensure the front leg is bent
• Keep both heels on the ground

Variations:
• A variation of the above is to have both legs straight, thereby stretching the gastrocnemius in both legs at the same time. The main limitation here is that one calf may be more flexible than the other.

Other Stretches

2. Unsupported upper calf stretch: (fig. 279)
Uses: This is a good position to flow into a lower calf stretch and hamstring stretch.
Description: Place one foot comfortably in front of the other and bend the front leg. With the upper body supported on the bent leg lean forwards. Keep the back leg straight and the heel on the floor.

Variations:
• In order to stretch the lower calf bend the back leg while keeping the upper weight on the front leg (fig. 280).
• Straighten the front leg and take the upper body weight on the bent back leg. Now reach forward and pull the toes of the straight leg towards the shin. During this stretch always ensure the upper weight is supported. (fig. 281).

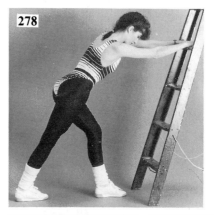

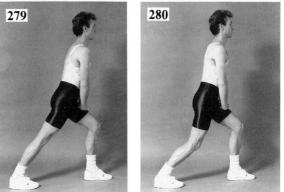

• Bring the heels together and bend both legs so the body is in a quarter squat. This will stretch the lower calves of both legs.

3. Seated straight leg calf stretch (fig. 282)
Uses: Stretches the gastrocnemius while also stretching the hamstrings and the lower back.
Description: Sit on the floor with one leg bent so the sole of the foot is against the knee of the straight leg. With the opposite hand on the straight leg, push down on the thigh and with the other hand pull the toes of the straight leg back. To increase the stretch on the hamstrings push down harder on the thigh.

Variations:
• With both legs together, stretch forward and pull the toes back ensuring that the head is up and the back is straight.
• With both legs together, contract the muscles of the front of the shins (tibialis anteria) so the foot is dorsi-flexed (fig. 283).

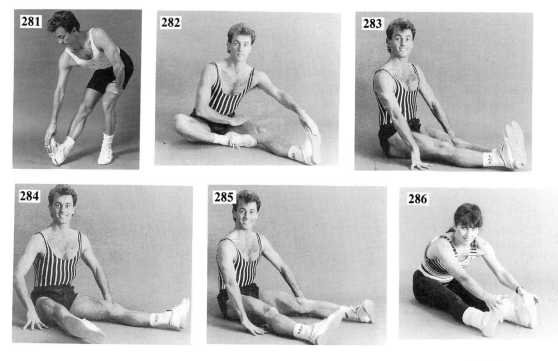

- To stretch gastrocnemius and the muscles around the ankle joint alternatively, turn the toes in and then out (figs. 284 and 285).

- To increase the stretch to the hamstrings and lower back while stretching the gastrocnemius and muscles around the ankle joint, lean forward and pull the feet inwards and then push them outwards (see figs. 286 and 287). Note that the body is in an unsupported forward flexed position (even though seated) so this stretch should not be held for more than 15 secs.

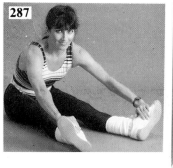

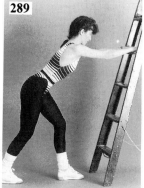

II Soleus

Standard Stretch

1. Standing bent leg calf stretch: (fig. 289)
Uses: Stretches the Soleus muscle. The soleus, like the gastrocnemius is used extensively in all explosive movements such as sprinting and jumping. It should be stretched, therefore, before and after most sports and activities.
Description: This stretches the lower part of the calf. The position for the stretch is the same as that for the standing straight leg calf stretch except that the back leg, like the front leg is also bent. To increase the stretch, lean forward but make sure the heel of the back leg remains on the ground.

Special considerations
- Same as for standing straight leg calf stretch.

Variations:
- A variation of the above is to have both legs bent. This will stretch the lower part of both calf muscles. The major concern with this variation is that one calf may be more flexible than the other.

Other stretches

2. Standing lower calf stretch
Uses: Stretches the soleus. This is a good position to commence some upper calf and hamstring stretches.
Description: Start with one leg in front of the other. Bend both legs and take the upper body weight on

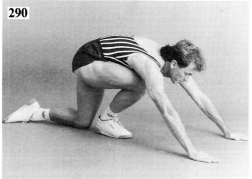

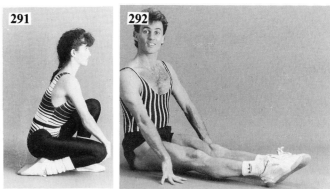

the front leg and move the hips forward. Ensure that the heel of the back leg is kept on the ground.

3. Kneeling lower calf stretch (fig. 290)
Uses: Stretches the soleus.
Description: Kneel on the floor and place the heel just in front of the opposite knee. Rest the chest on the knee and stretch forward while keeping the heel on the ground. **Ensure that the knee of the front leg is not in a hyperflexed position.**

III Tibialis Anterior

Standard stretch

1. Tibialis anterior bent leg stretch (fig. 291)
Uses: One of the few stretches that effectively stretches the tibialis anterior muscle. Poor flexibility of tibialis anterior can be the cause of anterior lower leg pain.
Description: Sit on the heel of one leg while supporting the upper body with the opposite hand. Now pull the knee up.

Special considerations
• While in this position the knee is in severe hyper-flexion so ensure that the total body weight is never on the heel.

2.2 Stretches for the Hip, Groin and Upper Leg

I Quadriceps

Standard stretch

1. Standing quadricep stretch (fig. 294)
Uses: The quadriceps have two primary actions; as a hip flexor and in lower leg extension. Tightness of the quadriceps can cause groin problems and

Other stretches

2. Tibialis anterior straight leg stretch (fig. 292)
Uses: Stretches the tibialis anterior by contracting the calf. This is also a good mobility exercise for the calf and shins during a warm-up.
Description: Sit on the floor with the legs straight. Point the toes away from the body. This exercise can be done alternatively with the stretches in figs 286 and 287.

Variations
• While in a seated position bend one leg and rest the ankle close to the knee. With the opposite hand pull the toes towards the body (fig. 293).

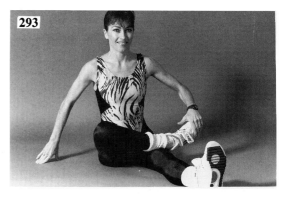

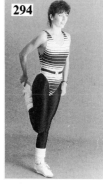

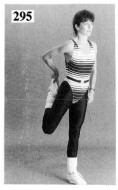

muscle tearing when participating in explosive movements such as sprinting. The standing quadriceps stretch is the standard exercise for maintaining flexibility of the quadriceps.

Description: Stand on one leg and pull the foot of the other leg into the buttock. Some people may have difficulty balancing on one leg. If this is the case, concentrate on something directly ahead or find a support such as a wall or stool. To increase the stretch, extend the hip (figure 295) and push the ankle against the resistance of the hand (i.e. as in a PNF stretch).

Variations
• Lateral quadricep stretch. The vastus lateralis can be effectively stretched by pulling the ankle towards the buttock of the leg that is not being stretched.
• Medial quadricep stretch. The vastus medialis can be stretched by pulling the ankle to the outside of the buttock of the leg being stretched.

Other stretches

2. Lying quadricep stretch (fig. 296)
Uses: A good alternative to the standing quadricep stretch.
Description: Lie on the stomach and pull the foot into the buttock. A variation is to pull the foot into the buttock with both hands (fig. 297). To increase the stretch, push the pelvis into the floor and slightly lift the thigh off the ground.

Variations
• **Side quadricep stretch.** Lie on one side and support the upper body on the arm. With the other hand, pull the foot into the buttock (figure 298). Ensure that the knees are together during this stretch.

3. Quadricep stretch using a stool or table (fig. 299)
Uses: Alternative quadricep stretch. In addition it

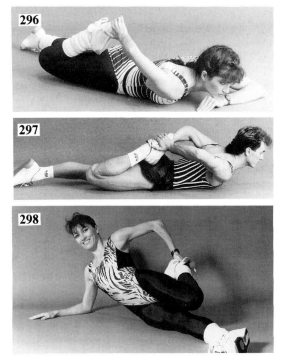

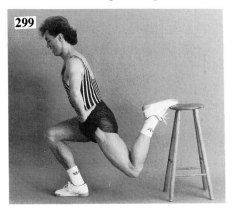

can be used in a sequence of stretches for the legs using a stool or table. (These are summarised later in this section.)
Description: With the leg bent, rest the foot on a stool. In order to stretch the quadriceps, bend the supporting leg.

II Hamstrings

Standard stretch

1. Standing hamstring stretch using a stool or table (fig. 300)
Uses: Stretches primarily biceps femoris of the hamstring group. The major action of the hamstrings is leg flexion with some hip extension.

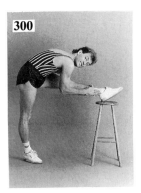
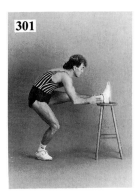

Runners are a group of athletes that are especially prone to either short or weak and tight hamstrings. However, most athletes should do some hamstring flexibility training while warming up and cooling down.

Description: With one leg straight, place the heel of the other leg on a stool. Bend with a straight back and hold the ankle of the leg that is on the stool. To increase the stretch, bend the arms and lower the chest to the thigh.

Special considerations:
• Always ensure the hamstrings have been warmed-up prior to stretching.
• If the hamstrings are exceptionally tight, slightly bend the knee of the leg being stretched.
• Always keep the back straight.

Variations:
• Same as the above but with the supporting leg bent (fig. 301).
• Same as the above except the hands grip the outside of the leg being stretched. This increases the stretch to the lower back and the medial portion of the hamstring group (fig. 302).
• For people with good hamstring flexibility, the leg being stretched can be lifted higher (fig. 303).

Other stretches

2. Seated hamstring stretch (fig. 304)
Description: Sit on the floor with both legs straight. Slowly bend forward from the hips and reach to the toes or ankles. To increase the stretch, bend the arms and lower the chest to the knees.

Special considerations:
• With poor flexibility, bend the knees slightly (fig. 305).
• Keep the head up.
• Don't arch the back but bend from the hips.

Variations:
• **Single leg seated hamstring stretch** (fig. 306). Sit

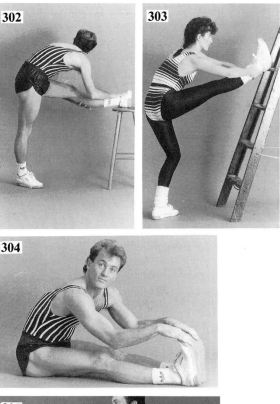

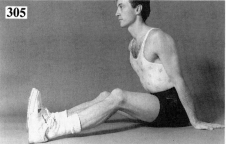

on the floor with one leg straight and the other bent so that the sole of the foot is touching the inside of the thigh. Bend forward and reach for the toes of the straight leg.

• **Single leg seated hamstring stretch** (fig. 307). Same as for figure 306 except the leg of the hamstring being stretched is bent.

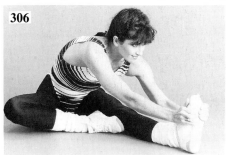

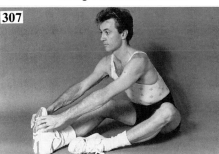

Potentially dangerous seated hamstring stretches

A common variation of the seated hamstring stretch which can be potentially dangerous is shown in figs 308 and 309. Here the bent leg is twisted to the side with the heel next to the buttock placing excessive pressure on the medial ligaments of the knee. The correct bent leg position is shown in figure 306.

3. Raised leg hamstring stretch (fig. 310)
Uses: Alternative hamstring stretch.
Description: Sit on the floor with both legs straight. Remain in a seated position and raise one leg, holding the sole of the foot. By pushing down against the hand the stretch becomes a PNF stretch. If the hamstrings are tight hold the ankle, not the foot and bend the other leg (fig. 311).

Variations:
• Lie on the back with both legs slightly bent. Hold the foot or ankle and pull towards the chest (fig. 312). Again, this stretch becomes a PNF stretch by resisting against the hands.

• Lie on the side and support the upper body with the elbow. Raise the top leg and pull the leg towards the shoulder (fig. 313). A PNF stretch can be incorporated by contracting the hamstrings against the resistance of the hand.

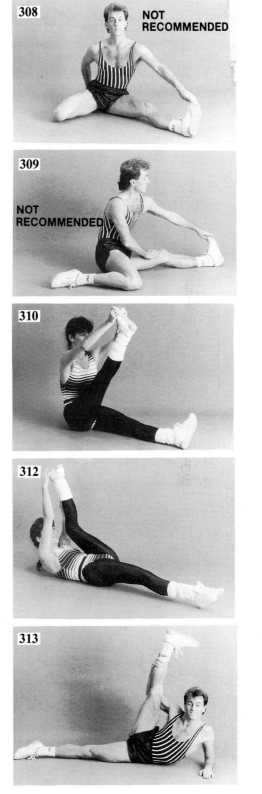

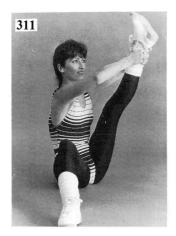

4. Kneeling hamstring stretch (fig. 314)

Uses: This is a good variation stretch from the seated hamstring stretch.

Description: From a kneeling position, straighten one leg (fig. 314). Ensure most of the body weight is on the hands. To increase the stretch, lower the chest towards the thigh of the straight leg.

5. Standing hamstring stretch (fig. 315)

Uses: This hamstring stretch is a good progression from the standing calf stretches (figs 279 and 280).

Description: While in a standing position, place one foot in front of the other. Keep the front leg straight and bend the back leg. Lean forward and take the weight of the upper on the bent leg.

III Abductor and Related Hip Muscles

Standard stretch

1. Hip flexor stretch (fig. 316)

Uses: This is a good stretch for superior portion of the quadriceps (hip flexors) and the deeper muscles of the hip (iliopsoas). If the iliopsoas is strengthened and not lengthened by stretching, extra strain can be put on the lumbar spine area resulting in lower back problems.

Description: Move one leg forward until the knee of the forward leg is directly over the ankle. The other knee should be resting on the floor. Without changing the position of the knee on the floor or the forward foot, lower the front of the hip to create a good stretch.

Variations:

• To increase the stretch, lean forward and while supporting the upper body weight (fig. 317).

Other stretches

2. Iliotibial band stretch (fig. 318)

Uses: Iliotibial band syndrome is a common injury suffered by joggers and distance runners. The symptoms are severe pain on the lateral condyle of the knee after about five minutes of running. The cause is tightening of the muscles that insert into the iliotibial band (e.g. gluteus maximus and tensor fasciae latae). Stretching the iliotibial band is one way of preventing and treating the problem.

Description: Place one leg forward. Bend forward and rest the chest on the bent knee. Now move the back leg so that it is under the superior portion of the thigh of the bent leg. To increase the stretch, drop the hip of the straight leg and support the body by placing the hands on the knees.

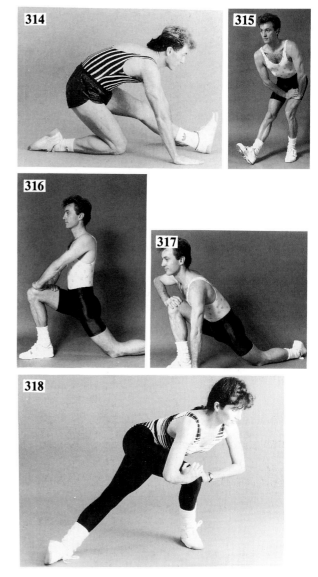

Variations:

• **Standing iliotibial band stretch.** Cross one foot over the other, twist around and look down towards the heel of the back leg (fig. 319). In order to increase the stretch, push the hip of the back leg out further. With the legs slightly apart (fig. 320) the stretch on the iliotibial band is reduced and the stretch on external obliques is increased.

• A wall or ladder can be effectively used to stretch the iliotibial band (fig. 321). Stand side-on to the wall and lean towards the wall with the hands above the head. Bend the inside leg and push the hip away from the wall.

• The stretch shown in fig. 322 is a good abductor stretch. Begin the stretch by kneeling on the floor

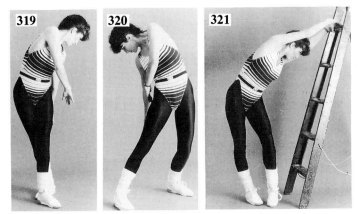

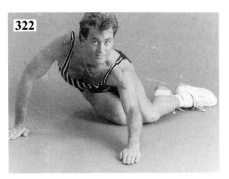

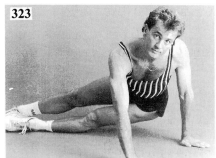

and drop one hip to the side while keeping the weight on the hands. A variation is to place the legs to the side, lift up with the hands and push the hips to the floor (fig. 323). This also stretches the external oblique muscle of the abdominal area.

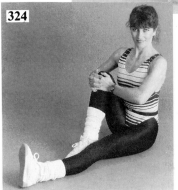

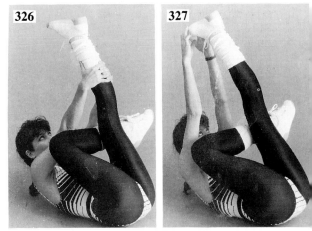

IV Gluteals

Standard stretch

6. Seated gluteals stretch (fig. 324)
Uses: The action of the gluteals is thigh extension, rotation and abduction. The gluteals are a powerful group of muscles that are used in just about all leg movements. There is a problem however in stretching them effectively.
Description: Sit on the floor with one leg straight and pull the other up to the chest with the hands. This same stretch can be done just as easily by sitting in a chair and pulling one knee to the chest.

Variations:
• **Advanced gluteal stretch** (fig. 325). Lie on the back. Bend both knees and place one ankle on the other knee. Now thread one hand between the legs, clasp the hands and pull the knee to the chest. This sounds awkward, but is an excellent isolation stretch for the gluteals.

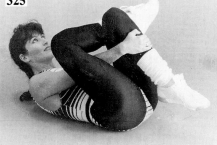

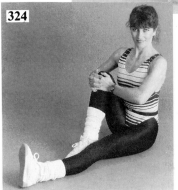

• By removing the hands from above the shin, and straightening the leg and pulling down on the ankle, the hamstrings are also stretched (fig. 326). In addition, the calf can be stretched by changing the position of the hands from the ankle to the toes (fig. 327).

• Lie on one side and support the trunk on the elbow, then bend the top leg and place the heel in front of the thigh (fig. 328). To increase the stretch pull the heel towards the trunk.

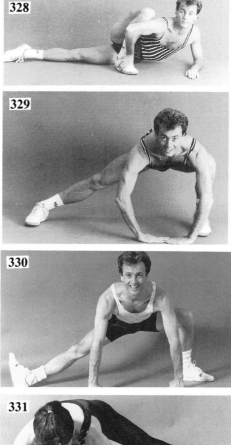

V Groin Adductor Stretches

Standard stretch

1. Classic adductor stretch (fig. 329)
Uses: The action of the groin adductors is, as the name suggests, powerful adduction of the thigh. In addition, they extend and rotate the thigh. Most sports and activities require severe groin adduction and if suppleness is poor in this area, there is a risk of injury.
Description: Lean forward and take the weight of the upper body on the hands. Move to the side by straightening one leg and bending the other. Make sure that the foot of the straight leg remains on the floor. To increase the stretch move more to the side and bend the arms so the shoulders are closer to ground.

Variations:
• as a progression from fig. 329, rotate the foot so that the heel takes the weight (fig. 330).

• by leaning forward and taking the weight on the forearms the adductors can be effectively stretched (fig. 331). It is important that the body weight is not taken on the supporting knee.

• sit on the floor and hold the soles of the feet together with one hand. Now, with the other hand on the inside of the leg, gently push down (fig. 332). This is a good isolation stretch of the groin.

• fig. 333 is an advanced adductor stretch that requires a certain amount of flexibilty. Lie on the stomach and place the soles of the feet together. To

increase the stretch move the knees further apart.
• fig. 334 is the reverse of fig. 333. Lie on the back and raise the bent legs in the air. Now pull the legs apart (at the thighs).

• fig. 335 is a progression of fig. 334. While on the back place the soles of the feet together and pull the ankles towards the body.

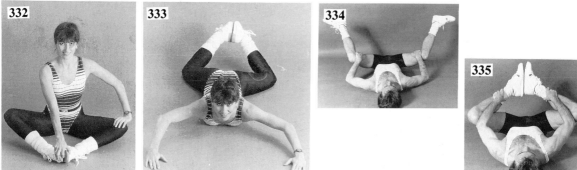

VI Adductor, Hamstring and Trunk Stretches

Standard stretch

Compound groin stretch (fig. 336)

Uses: A compound stretch that incorporates the groin adductors, hamstrings and lower back.

Description: Sit on the floor with the legs comfortably spread. Increase the stretch of the adductors by taking the weight of the body on the hands. Do this by placing one hand next to the buttocks and the other between the thighs. Lift the body up and move forwards while keeping the heels in the same spot. Now, lean forward and clasp the sole of the foot, or the ankle depending on the level of flexibility, with both hands. To increase the stretch on the hamstrings, lower the chest to the thigh, keep the head up and lean further forward. This can be incorporated into a PNF stretch by contracting the back muscles against the resistance of the hands.

Variations:

• Cross the hands over and clasp the foot or ankle (fig. 337). Incorporate a PNF stretch by contracting the back muscles against the resistance of the hands.

• To bring the upper back into the stretch, move the hands up and clasp the thigh (fig. 338). This reduces the stretch on the hamstrings but does not affect the adductor stretch. Incorporate a PNF stretch by contracting the upper back muscles against the resistance of the hands.

• For tight hamstrings and groin muscles place the hands behind the thighs and next to the buttocks (for support). Start with the legs bent (fig. 339) and as flexibility improves, straighten them (fig. 340).

• While in the same position as fig. 340, move one hand to the front twist to one side and lean forward (fig. 341).

• While in the same position as fig. 341, raise the front arm and stretch it above the head (fig. 342). The other arm is left behind the body to act as a support.

• As a progression from fig. 342 bend one leg and position the sole close to the thigh of the other leg.

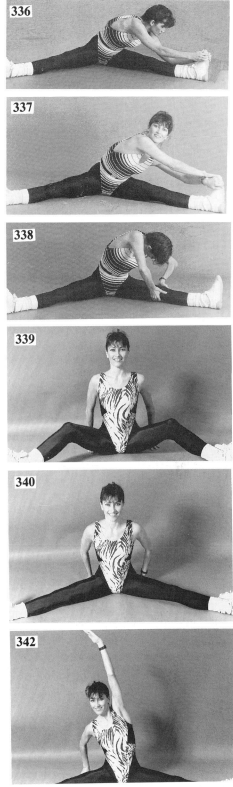

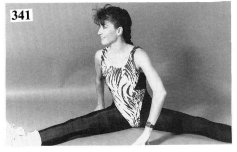

Now place the hand on the side of the head and lean to the side of the straight leg (fig. 343). Again it is important that the other arm is left behind the body to act as support.

• With legs bent and comfortably apart place the hands next to the buttocks for support. Now move the legs to one side and then the other (fig. 344).

2. Groin stretches using a stool or table (figs 345–6)
Uses: The following two stretches can be done using a ballet bar, stool, table, low wall etc. They are common stretches with runners who should carry them out in combination with calf, hamstring and quadricep stretches (figs 300 and 301).
Description: The first stretch (fig. 345) is basically the same as fig. 329, but here much of the upper body weight is supported by the stool. The second stretch (fig. 346), is an effective groin lower back stretch.

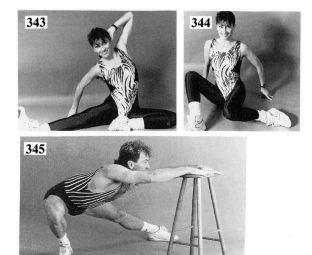

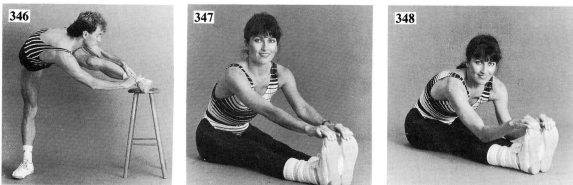

2.3 Stretches for the Lower Back and Trunk

I Lower back

Standard stretch

1. Seated toe touch (fig. 347)
Uses: The vertebral column is held together by strong ligaments and supported by muscles. With inactivity and ageing, the discs and ligaments may harden, leading to poor flexibility and eventually back pain. Specific stretching exercises for the lower back can help in preventing and alleviating back problems. The seated toe touch stretches the lower back muscles (inferior portion of erector spinae) that surround the lumbar vertebrae and hamstrings.
Description: Sit on the floor with legs straight and together. Lean forward by bending at the hips, *not the back*, and clasp the toes or ankles depending on the degree of flexibility (fig. 347). To increase the stretch, bend the arms and lower the chest to the

thighs (fig. 348). While in the fully flexed position a PNF stretch can be incorporated by trying to extend the back against the resistance of the hands.

Special considerations
• Do not stretch to the point of pain. Touching the toes or going further should only be considered a goal to be achieved.
• Do not bounce in and attempt to increase the stretch while in the fully flexed position.
• Do not bend forward with the back, but at the hips.

Variations:
• The stretch shown in fig. 349 is a variation of single leg seated hamstring stretch (fig. 306). Here, the wrists are crossed with the hands holding the feet or ankles. This can again be incorporated into

a PNF stretch by resisting against the hands.

• The stretch shown in fig. 350 is a good back stretch for those with poor hamstring flexibility. Spread the legs slightly so the heels or ankles can be comfortably held. Lean forward from the hips and pull with the arms. By resisting against the hands in the fully flexed position, a PNF stretch can be incorporated.

• Fig. 351 is a progression from figure 350 that isolates the back extensors on each side of the spine.

Other stretches

2. Knee to chest lower back stretch (fig. 352)
Uses: A very good exercise to loosen the lower back muscles and hamstrings.
Description: Lie on the back, clasp the hands around the knee and pull one leg to the chest. If possible, keep the back of the head on the floor and the other leg as straight as possible.

Variations:
• Lie on the back, clasp the hands around the sole of the foot and pull the knee to the chest. If possible keep the back of the head on the floor and the other leg straight.

• Lie on the back and bring one knee to the chest. Place the opposite hand on the bent knee and ease it over the thigh of the straight leg. Keep the shoulders on the ground and turn the face in the opposite direction to that of the bent knee (fig. 353).

• Lie on the back and bend both knees. Place one ankle on the lateral side of the other leg (fig. 354). Now pull the knee onto the floor with the other leg while ensuring the shoulders stay on the ground (fig. 355).

• Lie on the back with the arms spread. With the knees bent, flex the thighs and rotate them from one side to the other while keeping the shoulders on the floor (fig. 356).

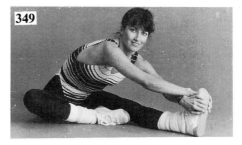

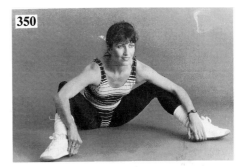

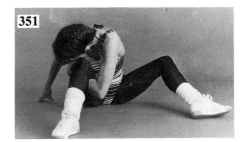

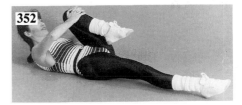

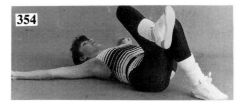

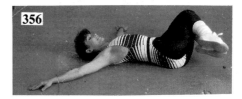

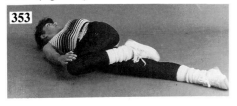

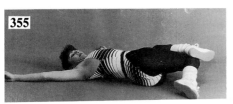

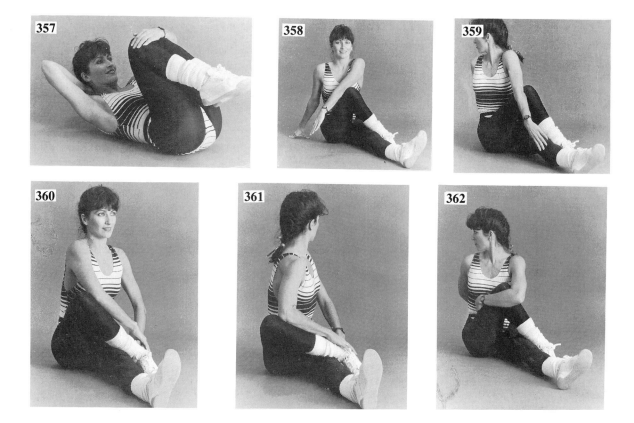

- Lie on the back with one hand behind the head. Bend the knees and pull them into the chest with the other arm (fig. 357).

3. Spinal twist (fig. 358)
Uses: The spinal twist is a good stretch for the upper back, lower back, side of the hips and rib cage. This stretch will help in rotation of the trunk.
Description: Sit on the floor with one leg straight. Bend the other leg and place the foot on the outside of the thigh of the straight leg (fig. 358). Now rotate the body and look over the shoulder of the arm that is supporting the body (fig. 359).

Variations:
- The stretch shown in fig. 360 stretches the hip rotators, adductor muscles and the lower back. Start the stretch by being in the same position as for fig. 358. Place the elbow closest to the bent knee, on the knee (fig. 360). Push down on the knee with the elbow and look over the opposite shoulder (fig. 361).
- The stretch shown in fig. 362 stretches the gluteals, hip adductors and lower back. Start the stretch by being in the same position as for fig. 358. Pull the bent leg into the chest with the forearm, rotate and look over the opposite shoulder (fig. 362).

4. Standing lower back stretch (fig. 363)
Uses: An effective stretch for the lower back and middle back which can easily be incorporated into a PNF stretch. It is very hard to stretch the back in a standing position due to the problems of forward flexion.
Description: With knees bent, bend over and cross the arms behind the knees (figure 363). Straighten the legs against the resistance of the arms and try and arch the back.

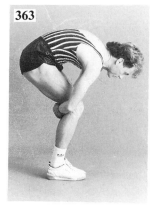

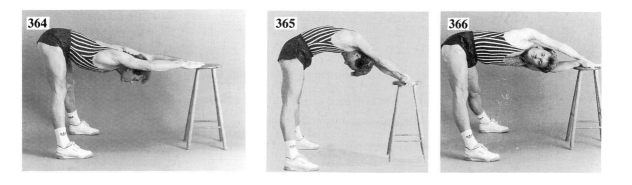

5. Hamstring, back and trunk stretch using a stool

Uses: By using a stool, table or chair as a support it is possible to stretch a number of different muscle groups at the same time. For example, it is possible to effectively stretch the hamstrings as well as the back and shoulders if the upper body is supported (fig. 364).

Description: Stand a comfortable distance from the stool and lean forwards and place the hands on the stool. While in this position lower the chest towards the floor to increase the stretch in the hamstrings, back and shoulders (fig. 364). Ensure the knees are not locked out.

Variations

• By arching the back upwards the emphasis of the stretch is changed to the middle portion of the back (fig. 365).

• By turning to one side and then the other the stretch takes the back through a rotational range of movement (fig. 366).

6. Standing lateral trunk stretch with support

Uses: To stretch the lateral trunk muscles, the muscles of the back and muscles of the chest.

Description: Stand side on to a wall or ladder and stretch the hands above the head. Lean sideways towards the ladder or wall (fig. 367). Make sure throughout the stretch that the front of the body is always at right angles to the wall.

Variations

• Fig. 368 shows the same stretch as fig. 367 except that a partner is being used as the support.

• Fig. 369 shows a good rotation stretch for the back. Stand close to a wall or ladder with the feet shoulder-width apart. Make sure that the feet remain on the floor and the twisting movement is slow and controlled and the stretch is held towards the end of range of movement.

• Fig. 370 shows the same stretch as fig. 369 except that a partner is being used as the support.

• Fig. 371 shows the same stretch as fig. 370 except that the hands are raised above the head thereby stretching the shoulders and the upper trunk muscles.

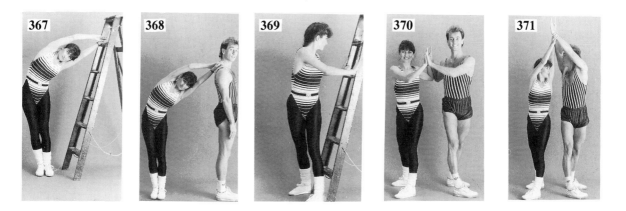

2.4 Stretches for the Upper Back and Neck

I Neck

Standard stretch

1. Neck range of movement stretches
(figs. 372–374)
Uses: There are six basic movements of the neck. These are:

- Neck flexion, or bending of the neck forwards
- Extension or bending backwards
- Side flexion to the left and right
- Rotation of the head to the right and left.

All of these movements can be stretched using a series of different stretches. The neck should *never* be stretched by a single rotation movement that takes it through its entire range of motion.

Description: Stand with the legs shoulder width apart, bend the head forward and then backwards (fig. 372). Continue the sequence of stretches by rotating the neck from left to right (fig. 373) and conclude by lowering the head to the left side and then to the right side (fig. 374). The direction for the above stretches can then be reversed.

Special considerations
- Treat the neck with extreme caution; do all the stretches slowly and comfortably.
- Never do complete neck rotations as this places extreme stress on the cervical vertebrae, especially in the extension phase.

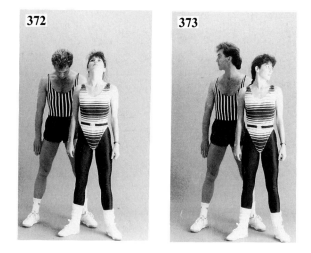

Variations
- A variation of the above sequence of neck stretches is to add some resistance in each direction. Start by clasping the hands behind the head and flex the head forwards (fig. 376), then place the hands on the forehead and extend the head backwards (fig. 377). Complete the sequence by placing one hand above the ear on the opposite side and lower the head to the shoulder (fig. 364). To increase this stretch reach down towards the knee with the opposite hand.

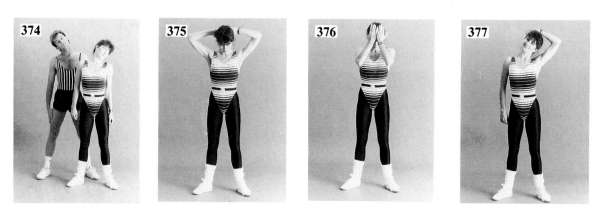

II Upper Back

Standard stretch

2. Cat stretch (fig. 378)

Uses: Stretches and mobilises the entire spine with special emphasis on the middle and upper back. In addition the cat stretch is excellent for improving posture.

Description: Crouch on all fours, raise the spine slowly upwards, then relax and let the stomach drop slowly. While doing this stretch concentrate on arching the upper spine.

Variations

• While crouching on all fours, stretch the left arm in front and the right leg out behind, then alternate the arms and legs.

• Stand with the feet shoulder-width apart, the knees slightly bent and cross the arms above the head. Now bend forwards, clasp the lateral side of the knees and pull up by arching the upper back (fig. 379).

Other stretches

3. Rolling back stretch (fig. 380)

Uses: Stretches and mobilises the muscles of the entire spine.

Description: This stretch is extremely uncomfortable if done on a hard surface. While in a sitting position hold the knees with the hands and pull them into the chest. Gently roll backwards so the body is resting on the spine. Now roll evenly backwards and forwards.

Special considerations

• Do not roll backwards to a point where pressure is put on the neck.

• Roll backwards and forwards evenly and with control—do not overdo it.

Potentially dangerous back exercise

• Fig. 381 shows a legs-overhead stretch called 'the plough'. Although this is common in yoga it is regarded as potentially dangerous because of the extreme load placed on the neck.

4. Upper back stretch (fig. 382)

Uses: Stretches the rhomboids, the opposing muscle to the 'pecs'.

Description: Stand with the legs bent and the feet shoulder width apart. Support the upper body with the hands on the thighs and spread the shoulder blades (fig. 382).

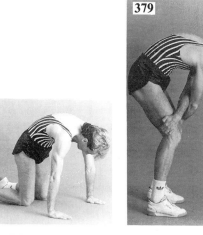

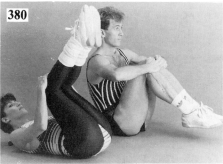

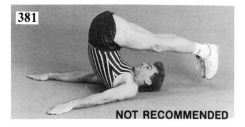

NOT RECOMMENDED

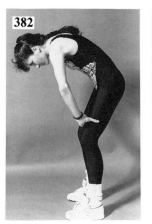

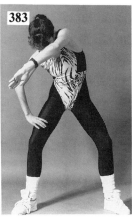

Variations:

• While in the same body position as for figure 382 take one hand off the thigh arm stretch the arm forward and across the body (fig. 383).

• Move into a sitting position and place the soles of the feet together. Place one hand behind the body for support and place the other hand on the opposite knee and pull gently (fig. 384).

• In order to stretch the latissimus dorsi muscle move into an all fours position. Place one hand next to the knee of the same side and position the other in front and in line with the head (fig. 385). To increase the stretch drop the shoulder of the extended arm.

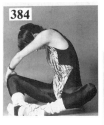

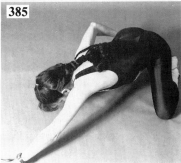

2.5 Stretches for the Shoulders, Arms and Chest

I Shoulders and Arms

Standard stretch

1. Standing shoulder stretch (fig. 386)
Uses: Stretches posterior muscles of the shoulder and the middle portion of the upper back. This is a good general stretch for most throwing activities and racket sports.
Description: Stand with the feet shoulder-width apart. Bend one arm and rest the hand on the opposite shoulder. Now, with the other hand pull the elbow towards the opposite shoulder. This stretch can incorporate a PNF stretch by contracting the posterior shoulder muscles against the resistance of the hand on the elbow.

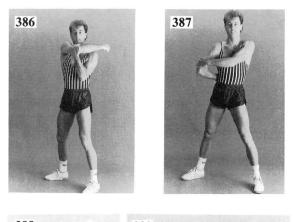

Variations

• Rest the back of one hand against the lumbar spine and pull the elbow of the other hand towards the front (fig. 387).

• Place one hand as far as possible down the back and if possible grasp the other hand that is positioned up the back and hold (fig. 388). Many people will be unable to get the hands to meet. If this is the case use a towel or piece of rope to bridge the gap between the hands.

• Fig. 389 is a good stretch for the triceps and other superior and posterior shoulder muscles. Place one hand down the back and push on the elbow with the other hand. Use the same position as fig. 389 but this time lean to one side to stretch the lateral trunk muscles (fig. 390). To increase the stretch push down harder on the elbow.

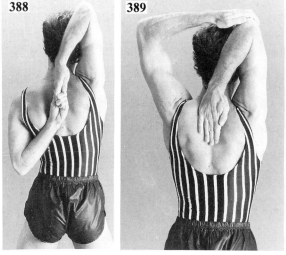

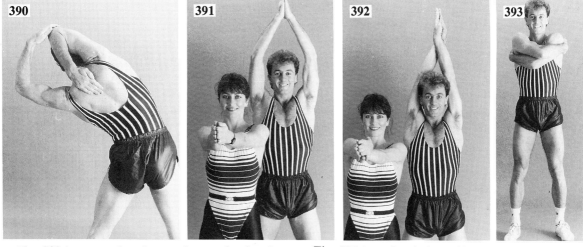

- Fig. 391 is more of an isometric exercise for the arms but it does stretch some of the muscle in the shoulders and the ribs. Start with the arms extended overhead and slightly backwards, stretch tall and squeeze the palms together, relax, lower the arms so they are straight out in front of the chest and squeeze again (fig. 391).

- Fig. 392 is an alternative to fig. 391 and is a great stretch for the outer portions of the arms, shoulders and ribs. Start with the arms extended overhead and slightly backwards. Cross the forearms and have the palms together (fig. 392) and stretch upwards while pushing the palms together. Relax, lower the arms so they are straight out in front of the chest and squeeze again (fig. 392).

- Fig. 393 stretches the shoulder and upper back muscles. Cross the arms in front of the body, place the hands on the shoulders and squeeze.

- Fig. 396 is a simple but effective stretch for the anterior shoulder muscles and also the muscles of the chest. With the feet shoulder width apart and the legs slightly bent, clasp the hands behind the back and push the arms back while keeping them straight.

- The stretch shown in fig. 394 starts by stretching the anterior shoulder muscles and chest muscles and then with only a slight change it stretches the posterior shoulder muscles and upper back muscles. Start by placing the palms of the hands in the small of the back (lumbar area) and try to bring the elbows together (*see* fig. 394). To change the stretch try to bring the elbows to the side.

- Fig. 395 is a simple but effective shoulder stretch. Simply have one arm straight out in front and the other bending and stretch by reaching forwards and backwards at the same time.

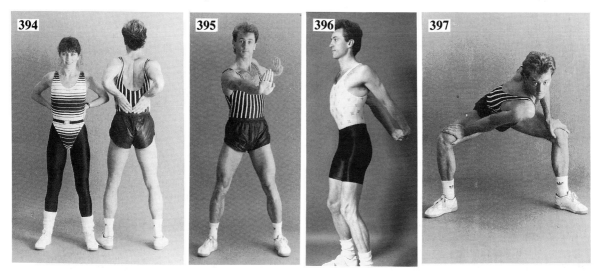

- Fig. 397 is a good compound stretch that stretches the shoulders, lateral trunk muscles, the lower back and the groin. Start the stretch with the feet slightly wider than shoulder-width apart, the legs bent and the hands resting on the knees. Now, straighten one arm and push down on the knee, while at the same time bending the other arm.

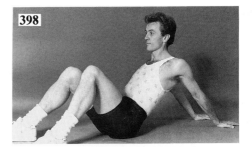

- Fig. 398 stretches the same muscle as in figure 394. This is a good shoulder stretch when on the floor. While seated with the legs bent place the hands behind the back and move the buttocks forward.

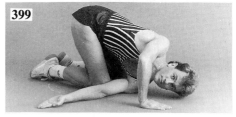

- Fig. 399 is often referred to as 'threading the needle' and is an effective spine and shoulder stretch. Start on all fours and thread one arm through the space between the supporting arm and the knee. To increase the stretch, lower the shoulder closer to the floor and reach out with the arm.

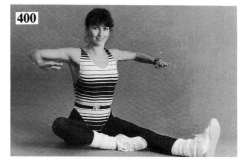

- Fig. 400 shows a groin, hamstring and shoulder stretch. Sit on the floor with one leg straight and the other bent so that the sole of the foot is next to the inside of the knee. Bend the arms as in fig. 400 and stretch the elbows back. Many of the previous shoulder stretches such as those in figs 386–93 can be done in this seated position.

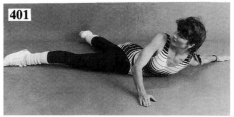

- Fig. 401 is a good cool-down stretch for the shoulders and upper back. Lie on the floor face down with the legs slightly spread and the arms out to the side. Push up with one arm and look over the same shoulder.

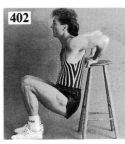

- Fig. 403 is an example of how the shoulders can be stretched using a stool or table. Gently lower the body until the stretch is felt in the shoulders.

Other stretches

2. Wrist and finger stretch (figs 403–4)

Uses: Maintains the range of movement of the muscles in the forearm that are responsible for wrist flexion and extension.

Description: Flex the arm as shown in fig. 386 and slowly flex and extend the fingers individually. In order to stretch the wrist, flex it forward and then press down on it with the other hand fig. 403). In order to stretch the wrist in extension, simply reverse the procedure for wrist flexion (fig. 404).

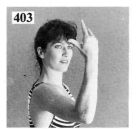

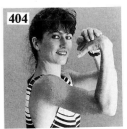

2.6 Partnership PNF Stretches

A PNF stretch is any stretch where the muscle is statically stretched, isometrically contracted against an immovable resistance, and then statically stretched again. Many of the individual stretches described in this section can incorporate the PNF principle of stretching. However PNF stretching is much more effective when done in a controlled situation with a partner.

Outlined below are examples of different PNF stretches, for the legs/hips, the lower back/trunk, the shoulders and neck. The only limit to the number of different PNF stretches that can be done is one's imagination.

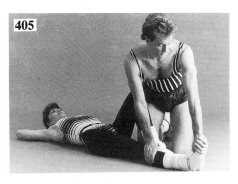

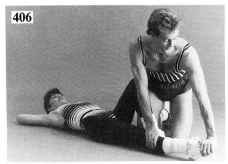

I PNF Stretches for the Legs and Hips

1. Tibialis anterior stretch (fig. 405)
Uses: Lengthens and strengthens the major muscle at the front of the lower leg that dorsi-flexes the foot. A good stretch for preventing and treating shin splint problems.
Description: Lie on the back with one leg bent and the other straight. Point the foot (plantar flexion) of the straight leg. Now isometrically dorsi-flex the foot against the resistance provided by a partner who has one hand on the shin and the other on the foot. Hold for 6–10 seconds, relax, then take the muscle into further stretch.

2. Gastrocnemius stretch (fig. 406)
Uses: Stretches the calf muscle.
Description: Sit on the floor with one leg bent and the other straight. Dorsi-flex the foot of the straight leg. Now isometrically plantar-flex the foot against the resistance provided by a partner. Hold for 6–10 seconds, relax, then move further into the stretch.

3. Hamstring stretch (figs 407–409)
Uses: Stretches the hamstring group of muscles,

namely: biceps femoris, semitendinosus and semimembranosus.
Description: Lie on the back with one leg straight on the floor and the other raised in the air. The partner kneels and rests the extended leg on the shoulder (fig. 407). Now isometrically contract the hamstrings against the resistance of the partner. Relax, statically stretch the hamstrings to a new point of reference and isometrically contract again (fig. 408).

Variation
• The partner can also include a PNF calf stretch by placing some resistance on the sole of the top of the foot (fig. 409).

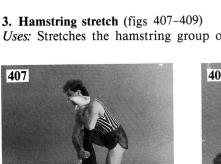

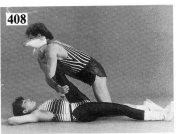

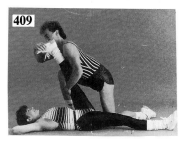

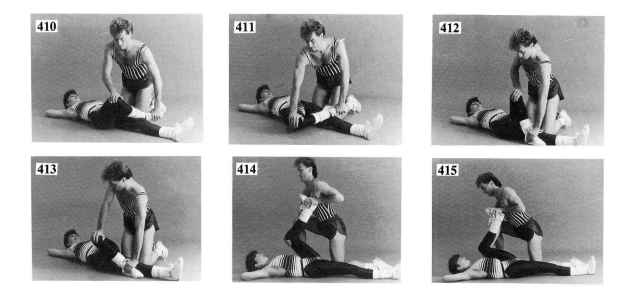

4. Hip adductor and internal rotator stretch
(figs 410–11)

Uses: Stretches the hip adductor muscles and to a lesser extent the internal rotators.

Description: Lie on the back with one leg straight and the other bent and with the lateral part of the ankle resting on the knee of the straight leg (fig. 410). Now isometrically contract the hip adductors against the resistance of the partner. Relax, statically stretch the adductors to a new reference point and isometrically contract again (fig. 394).

5. Hip abductor and external rotator stretch
(figs 412–13)

Uses: Stretches the hip abductor muscles and to a lesser extent the external rotators.

Description: Lie on the back with one leg straight and the other bent so that the lateral malleolus of the ankle is next to the lateral condyle of the knee (fig. 412). Now isometrically contract the hip abductors against the resistance of the partner. Relax, statically stretch the hip abductors to a new point of reference and isometrically contract again (fig. 411).

6. Hip extensor stretch (figs 414–15)

Uses: Stretches the hip extensor muscles such as gluteus maximus and the hamstrings.

Description: Lie on the back with one leg straight and the knee of the other leg bent at 90 degrees. Flex the hip so that the bent knee is close to the chest (fig. 414). Now isometrically contract the hip extensors against the resistance of the partner. Relax, statically stretch the hip extensors to a new point of reference and isometrically contract again (fig. 415).

7. Hip flexor stretch (figs 416–17)

Uses: Stretches iliopsoas, rectus femoris and other minor hip flexor muscles.

Description: Lie on the stomach with both legs straight. Extend one leg and isometrically contract the hip flexors against the resistance of the partner (fig. 412). Relax, statically stretch the hip flexors to

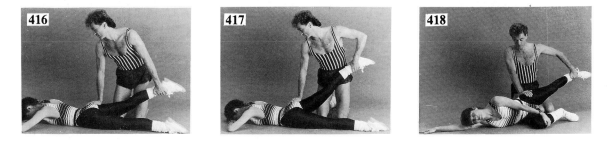

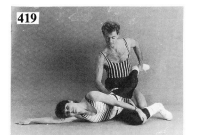

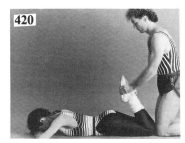

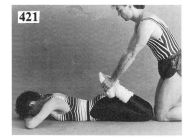

a new reference point and isometrically contract again (fig. 417).

Variation
• Lie on the side with the bottom leg bent and the top leg straight. Extend the hip of the straight leg and isometrically contract the hip flexors against the resistance of the partner (fig. 418). Relax, statically stretch the hip flexors to a new reference point and isometrically contract again (fig. 419).

8. Lower leg extensor stretch (figs 420–1)
Uses: Stretches the quadricep muscles, namely: rectus femoris, vastus lateralis, vastus medialis and vastus intermedius.
Description: Lie on the stomach and flex the lower leg at the knee by bringing the heels to the buttocks. Isometrically contract the quadriceps against the resistance of the partner (fig. 420). Statically stretch the quadriceps to a new reference point and isometrically contract again (fig. 421).

II PNF Stretches for the Lower Back and Trunk

1. Lower back stretch (figs 422–3)
Uses: Stretches the erector spinae and quadratus lumborum muscles—both of which are back extensors.
Description: Sit on the floor with the legs bent and comfortably spread. Hold the ankles and bend forwards at the hips (not the back). Isometrically contract the back extensor muscles against the resistance of the partner (fig. 422). Statically stretch forwards to a new reference point and isometrically contract again (fig. 423).

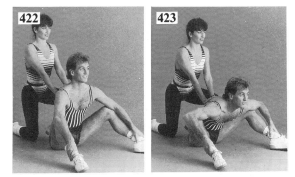

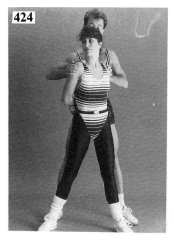

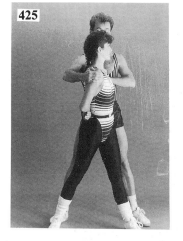

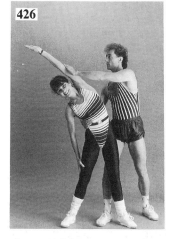

2. Trunk rotator stretch (figs 424–5)
Uses: Stretches the internal and external obliques,

erector spinae and other trunk rotator muscles.
Description: Stand with the feet shoulder width

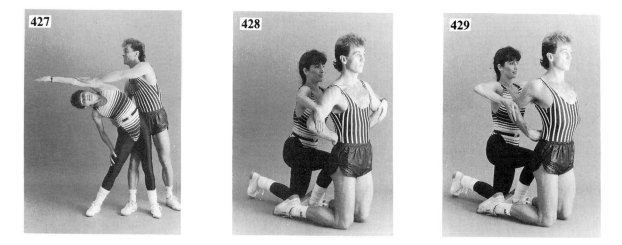

apart and the hands crossed behind the back. Rotate to one side while keeping the hips facing to the front. Isometrically contract the trunk rotators against the resistance of the partner (fig. 424). Rotate the trunk to a new reference point and isometrically contract again (fig. 425).

3. Lateral trunk stretch (figs 426–27)
Uses: Stretches the lateral trunk muscles from the obliques to the shoulder adductors.
Description: Stand with the feet shoulder-width apart. Place one hand on the thigh and the other arm above the head. Flex the trunk to the side that has the hand on the thigh (make sure the trunk is correctly aligned). Isometrically contract the lateral trunk muscles against the partner who has one hand around the waist and the other on the upper arm (fig. 426). Flex the trunk further to a

new reference point and isometrically contract (fig. 427).

III PNF Stretches for the Shoulders

1. Shoulder stretches
Uses: The following stretches stretch the muscles involved in shoulder flexion, extension, abduction, adduction, medial and lateral rotation.
Descriptions: **Shoulder flexion and adduction stretch.** This stretch also includes the medial rotators of the shoulders. Kneel on the floor with the hands on the hips. Extend the shoulders back (fig. 428) and isometrically contract the shoulder flexors and adductors against the resistance of the partner. Statically stretch the shoulder flexors and adductors and isometrically contract them again (fig. 429).

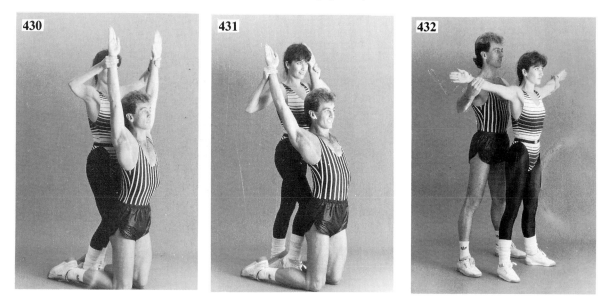

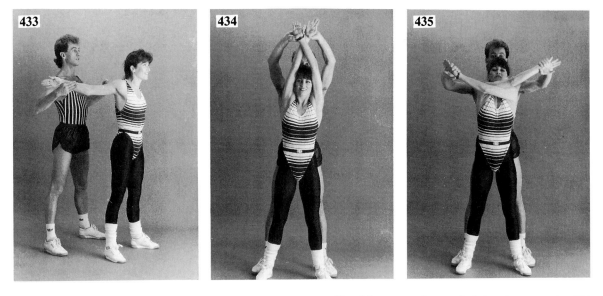

433 434 435

Variations
• The stretches shown in figs 430–1 are shoulder extension stretches that can be used in progression from fig. 429.

• The stretches shown in figs 432–3 are also a variation of the above. With the arms spread wide, the levers become longer and as such, the partner should be careful not to forcefully pull the arms back during the static stretch.

• **Shoulder extension and abduction stretch.** This stretch also includes the lateral rotators of the shoulders. Stand with the feet shoulder-width apart and the hands above the head (fig. 434). Keep the arms straight and cross them in front of the head. The partner may assist by gently pulling the arms down. Isometrically contract the muscles against the resistance of the partner. Statically stretch the shoulders further and then isometrically contract the muscles again (fig. 435).

IV PNF Stretches for the Neck

1. Neck stretches
Uses: Stretches the neck in flexion, extension, side flexion, and left and right rotation. These stretches can be done very effectively with or without a partner.

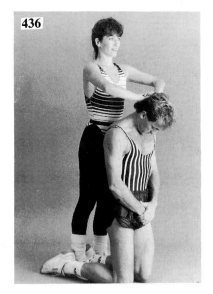

436

Variations
• **Neck flexion.** Kneel on the floor and flex the neck forwards into a static stretch. Isometrically contract against the resistance of the partner (fig. 419). Relax and repeat.

• **Neck extension.** Same as for fig. 436 except extend the head back.

• **Side neck flexion.** Same as for fig. 436 except flex the neck to the side.

• **Neck rotation.** Same as for fig. 436 except rotate the neck to the side.

References

Anderson, B., *Stretching*, Shelter Publications, California, 1980

Balaskas, B. & Stirk, J., *Soft Exercise. The Complete Book of Stretching*, Unwin Paperbacks, Sydney, 1983

Benyo, R., *Indoor Exercise Book*, Runner's World Books, California, 1981

Carter, V. (ed), *The Perfect Fitness Book*, Octopus Books Ltd and Womens Day, Australia, 1979

Cohen, H. (ed), *The Complete Encyclopedia of Exercises*, Paddington Press, USA 1979

Crouch, J., *Functional Human Anatomy*, Lea & Febiger, Philadelphia, 1970

Cullum, R., *YMCA Guide To Exercise To Music*, Pierson, Sydney, 1986

Dominguez, R. & Shyne, K., *To Stretch or Not to Stretch*, The Physician & Sports Medicine, 10(9), 1982

Editors of Consumer Guide, *Exercising Together*, Beekman House, New York, 1981

 Aerobic Dancing, Beekman House, New York, 1979

 Stretching for Shaping and Fitness, Beekman House, New York, 1981

Egger, G., *Common Sense Health*, Allen and Unwin, Sydney, 1986

Egger, G. & Champion, N., *The Fitness Leader's Handbook*, 3rd edition, Kangaroo Press, Sydney, 1989

Ellix, T., *Aerobic Fitness*, Greenhouse, Melbouren, 1986

Epley, B., *Dynamic Strength Training For Athletes*, Wm C. Brown, Iowa, 1985

Fox, E., *Sports Physiology*, W.B. Saunders, Philadelphia, 1979

Getchell, B., *Physical Fitness A Way Of Life*, John Wiley and Sons, New York, 1981

Hay, J., *The Biomechanics of Sports Techniques*, Prentice Hall, Inc., Englewood Cliffs, N.J., 1973

Holt, L.E., *Scientific Stretching For Sport*, Dalhousie University, Halifax, 1974

Howell, R. & Howell, M., *Foundations of Physical Education*, William Brooks, Queensland, 1984

Jones, A., *Nautilus Training Principles*, Medical Ind., Florida, 1971

Kennedy, R., *Beef It! Upping the Muscle Mass*, Sterling Publishing Co., Inc., New York, 1985

Lamberti, I., *Pumping Iron Without Pain*, Leisure Press, New York, 1983

Main, S., *Fit All Over: A Complete Catalogue of Exercises*, 3 S Fitness Group, California, 1984

Mirkin, G., *The Sports Medicine Book*, Paul Hamlyn Pty Ltd, Sydney, 1979

Pearl, B., *Keys To the Universe*, Physical Fitness Architects, California, 1982

Pyke, F. (ed), *Towards Better Coaching*, AGPS, Canberra, 1980

Shmidtbleicher, D., *Strength Training Part 1: Classification of Methods*, Science Periodicals on Research & Technology in Sport, W-4, August, 1985

Thompson, C., *Manual of Structural Kinesiology*, Times Mirror/Mosby College Publishing, St Louis, 1985

Watson, P., *The Muscle Maintenance Manual*, Kangaroo Press, Sydney, 1983

Weider, J., *The Best of Joe Weider's Muscle and Fitness: Training Tips and Routines*, Contemporary Books, Inc., Illinois, 1981

Index